MW01233410

Bittersweet Chances

A Personal Journey of Living and Learning in the Face of Illness

by

Dana Selenke Broehl

PublishAmerica
Baltimore

First printing

About the Cover

The artwork for the book's cover was painted by my husband. The angel represents the gift of life that ultimately came from God, and the two wings represent Doug's new lungs. The angel appears peaceful yet somber; she represents the bittersweet nature of life.

Special thanks to Nathan Chow for his artistic vision and layout design of the cover.

ISBN: 1-4137-1324-6
PUBLISHED BY PUBLISHAMERICA, LLLP
www.publishamerica.com
Baltimore

Printed in the United States of America

This book is dedicated to my husband, Doug, who gave me my first bittersweet chance when he proposed. It is also dedicated to all of the doctors and nurses who have cared for him over the years and understand the concept of bittersweet chances better than anyone. In particular, I would like to acknowledge Dr. Elaine Mischler, Dr. Guillermo do Pico, Dr. Julie Biller, and Mary Ellen Freeman for their years of compassionate care. And finally, this journey would not have been possible without the gift of life from Doug's donor and family. Doug and I are eternally grateful.

Acknowledgements

I would like to acknowledge the following friends and family for their invaluable support and love during this journey.

Glenda Selenke—Thank you for the endless supply of unconditional love, support, and laughter. I know that you were there in spirit.

Donnie Selenke—You were my one and constant presence. I'm so grateful for the time that we had together. You amazed me. Don't be afraid to show that side—it's too good to hide.

Mike Selenke—Thanks for being my big brother and trying to protect me from the big bad world. You are my one and only sarcasm twin. I will always remember our laughter and immaturity: "It tastes like home" and the fuzzy buzzy.

Chuck Broehl—Thank you for your support, and thank you for raising such a wonderful and resilient son. I wish Pat were here to see her son breathe again.

Lisa German—Here's to the sister I never had. Thanks for being everyone's protector and guardian angel.

Karen Keane Lazar—To the best friend a girl could ever ask for. You are a jewel, and I treasure you more than you will ever know. And Dan, Karen couldn't ask for a better husband.

Mr. Bill Keane—Thank you for your baby-sitting skills. You are a tremendous man, and I have always admired your patience and self-less nature. God bless you.

Brenda Karls and Ellen Lehman—Special thanks to my road trippers and ass amigas. You were lifesavers.

Amy Wentworth—Thanks for taking such good care of Willy and my students. Willy thanks you too. "Meow, meow."

Jeff Schalk—Thanks for the entertainment. The raw 'roo and the sweaty upper lip still make me laugh.

Be kind, for everyone you meet is fighting a battle.

—John Watson

Some people grumble because roses have thorns. I am thankful that thorns have roses.

—Karr

Contents

Introduction

"I have a disease called cystic fibrosis." At the time in which my future husband spoke those words to me, I had no idea how profoundly and dramatically his disease would alter the course of my life. In retrospect, I now realize that it was at that moment that his disease became my disease and my reality. As a result, the moment in which those words were uttered became a strangely difficult but cherished memory of my life. Those words changed me, but nothing altered my reality and view of the world so utterly and completely like the unexpected phone call in which I heard my simultaneously terrified and excited husband proclaim, "They might have new lungs for me."

I watched cystic fibrosis slowly and methodically devour my husband until he was given a second chance at life by way of a double lung transplant. During the course of his transplant and hospital stay, I kept family, friends, and members of our two online support groups updated through daily journal style emails. As a result, several people encouraged me to share those emails and my experiences in the form of a book. So it is through that encouragement that I have made a decision to open my very personal and private world of joy, sadness, and growth.

I do not proclaim to be Socrates, although I do fear that I will one day look like him as I approach middle age and my estrogen levels begin to wane. But I digress. My hope is that all individuals will be able to see and savor the profound beauty of life irrelevant of its circumstances. At some point, we will all face our mortality or the mortality of a loved one, and we will forever be altered.

If you have yet to have this experience, this book will encourage you to look at the beauty of your charmed life. If you are in the midst of this experience, this book will encourage you to look at the beauty of your charmed life. If this experience is now a cataloged memory in your psyche, this book will encourage you to look at the beauty of your charmed life. Are you getting my point?

No matter what our circumstances, no matter how profoundly sweet or how profoundly sour life is, there is beauty in everything. In fact, there is often more beauty and more opportunity for growth and self-awareness in those experiences that we deem as unpleasant or difficult. Embrace the difficult and see the lessons to be learned, and you will grow in unimaginable ways.

If all difficulties were known at the outset of a long journey, most of us would never start out at all.

—Dan Rather

The Beginning of the Journey

I met Doug on July 3, 1994, we were engaged on March 17, 1995, and we were married on October 28, 1995. "Boy, that seems a bit fast," I hear you say. Oh my, you have absolutely no idea just how fast it was for this shy and conservative former Catholic schoolgirl from Kansas.

I had never been boy crazy, and quite honestly, I had almost always viewed most men as a nuisance. I spent my prime dating years with my nose in a book and hanging out with girlfriends, and that was more than enough to make me happy. Men, I thought, were pleasant enough creatures, but I just couldn't imagine ever being able to find a guy who didn't scratch himself, delight in bodily functions, or watch sports endlessly. I had no scientific proof, but high levels of testosterone did seem to short-circuit the male brain.

If I were to ever consider a relationship, I decided that I would settle for no less than a Renaissance man: someone who enjoyed the finer things in life like reading, movies, music, and art. I also wanted a man who had the capacity and desire to engage in thoughtful and meaningful conversation. What I wanted, I mused, was a gay guy who liked girls. But I gave little thought to men, and I decided that if a relationship were in my future, it would just happen. With that philosophical approach to relationships, I frankly had a better chance of being hit in the head by a meteor. But I was a young and ignorant girl who thought that she understood the world much better than she actually did.

After graduating from college, I immediately began teaching at Kettle Moraine, a suburban Milwaukee high school that is tucked among some of Wisconsin's many beautiful and rolling glacial hills. I was elated to have a job and a paycheck, and I couldn't wait to make my mark on my students and the teaching world. But the only marks that were made during my first year of teaching were reflected in the bruises that littered my disappointed ego. Seasoned teachers often refer to the first year of teaching as a trial by fire. My first year of teaching was a trial by blazing inferno.

I quickly became consumed with my work, and I delighted in working myself to the point of exhaustion. I was a consummate perfectionist, and I would agonize over and rework every project, worksheet, and activity in a bizarre quest for some sort of master teacher perfection. But despite all of my best efforts and hard work, I would return home every evening feeling the same sense of dissatisfaction with my teaching ability. I ultimately knew that my students were learning, but I always felt that I could be doing more or doing better. The complexity and difficulties of my new job were completely overwhelming to me, and I was ignorant enough to believe that the only solution to my dissatisfaction was to work harder.

In addition to trying to master the art of teaching my subject matter, I was also attempting to play the part of counselor, social worker, and confidant in the lives of many of my students and their parents. I was always befuddled when forty-year-old parents would sit across from my desk and seek my counsel. Did they honestly expect me to know all of the answers? I would pretend to be wise and dispense advice, but I was really quite clueless. I was constantly plagued by a desire to turn around and search for the person to whom they were speaking. Was Gandhi, Jesus, or Yoda standing behind me? I was only twenty-two years old, and my life experience was so limited. I was born and raised in Kansas, and I had spent my teenage years in Wisconsin. I knew about wheat, The Wizard of Oz, cheese, and snow. I had traveled to Europe and Central America, but these experiences did little to help me solve the problems of frustrated parents who were trying to unravel the mysteries of teenage angst and volatility.

I felt much too young and naïve for the role of a teacher, and my disillusionment grew to resemble a virulent super strain of the Ebola virus: it was raging out of control and replicating at an incalculable and unmanageable rate. I began to wonder if I had chosen the wrong profession. I was just too young to feel so old, clueless, and tired. I seriously contemplated leaving the profession, but I refused to fail, and I made a decision to return for a second year.

My second year was much smoother, but I continued to be plagued by many of the same problems and challenges. I finally began to enjoy teaching, and I knew that I was growing professionally, but I had yet to learn the art of balancing work with fun. For me, being a successful teacher still meant being completely devoted to my craft to the point of insanity. I continued to obsess over every lesson, create hand-made bulletin boards monthly, and worry incessantly about students who were difficult or challenging.

This insanity eventually led to chronic fatigue and sporadic illnesses for which I refused to stay home. I was just completely unable or unwilling to see how out of control my life had become, and I was destined to continue down this path until something stopped me and brought me to my senses. There was a wake up call in my future, and it came in the form of a car crash.

In the fall of 1992, I had been sick for days, but I refused to stay home. There was only one day remaining before the Thanksgiving break, and I reasoned that I could tough out one more day before the short vacation. It was a gray and cold day, and it had just started to snow before I left my apartment. During the short drive to work, the snow began to increase in intensity, but I paid little attention to it. I was already in teacher mode, and I was running through the lessons for the day. As I began to drive up a hill, I could feel my car begin to slide, and before I knew it, I had crossed the centerline and was in the oncoming lane. My life was about to be irrevocably and beautifully altered by a bright flash of light, a jarringly intense jolt, and the sound of grinding metal.

When my car came to a stop, I found myself in a ditch. My car was white, and I was surrounded by the white snow that continued its silent and methodic cascade to earth. Everything was white, and I began to wonder if I was in the proverbial tunnel of white light. Go to the light, Dana. Go to the light. But why could I hear Michael Jackson's song "Black or White"? Was heaven a never ending Michael Jackson concert? Dear God, please let me go to hell.

But I was not dead. I was a lucky young woman who was listening to a pop radio station in a crushed car. I was momentarily hypnotized by the music that continued to blare from the car's radio, my inability to comprehend what had just happened, and my inability to believe that I was still alive. I searched my body for missing appendages, and when I had concluded that all of my body parts were still intact and functioning, I quickly climbed out of the passenger's side, walked up and out of the ditch, and re-entered my life.

I was taken by ambulance to the hospital, but my physical injuries were very minor. The emotional injuries, however, were slightly more pronounced and would provide the impetus that would help me to begin to make changes in my life.

I had never given much thought to my own mortality until I had the car wreck. I had always reasoned that death was for people who were either sick or old, and since I was young and healthy, death was not a part of my world or reality. But the accident allowed me to understand that death was an equal opportunity employer; health, vitality, and age were inconsequential in death's eyes.

Blessed with my new understanding of death and the fragility of my own life, I began to analyze my life in ways that I never had. I began to wonder if I could have been content with my life if I had lost it on that gray and snowy day. The answer was a resounding and deafening, "No!"

I knew immediately that I needed to make some serious and immediate changes in my life. To begin, I knew that I needed to stop relying on my job for satisfaction and happiness. My job was just a job; it was not and could not be responsible for my personal well-being. I was responsible for my own happiness, and for the first time in my life, I began to consider the possibility of marriage. I discovered that having a long-term relationship with someone was something that I wanted, if not craved. I wanted to open myself to the possibility of a romantic relationship. I wanted to love, and I wanted to be loved.

Most importantly, I discovered that I needed to rekindle my distant and neglected relationship with God. I had grown up Catholic, and I had attended a Catholic grade school, high school, and college. However, I had grown restless with the religion, and I slowly and progressively drifted away from it. For me, there was no joy in Catholicism; there was only fear and guilt. God felt distant and unknowable. I treasured the seeds of faith that the Catholic Church had given me, but I wanted and needed more joy in my faith. As a result, I walked away from the Catholic Church, but I never sought the shelter and comfort of a different church. And although I never abandoned my relationship with God, I put him on the back burner along with everything else of substance in my life. I chose to neglect the reality that I needed him to be a complete presence in my life if I were to have any sense of harmony and balance.

The car wreck and the emotional awakening that resulted would allow me to reprioritize my life and achieve the balance that I had lost. I had been slow to learn what truly mattered in life, and I was not going to blow this God given opportunity.

The changes in my life began immediately. I quit changing bulletin boards every month, I refused to do more than an hour or two of school work at home, I started attending services at a small Presbyterian church a few miles from my apartment, and I began to date again. Life was easier, and I finally felt the balance and harmony that had eluded me for so long. I began to savor the pure sweetness of my life, and it was good—very good.

Despite all of the changes that I had implemented in my life, dating continued to be my most daunting challenge. After a few lackluster attempts at the dating scene, I finally decided that I would join a dating service. Good grief, had I become this desperate? I wrestled with decision for several months, and I silently wondered if I were a complete and utter loser. Was this to be my fate? Would I be destined to date men who played Nintendo and lived in their parents' basement, or would I be destined to be a spinster surrounded by her forty cats and baskets of knitting needles?

My friends were more than encouraging about this new dating prospect for me, but I knew that they were just anxious to see some poor old sap actually join a dating service. I knew that I would just be a tremendous source of entertainment for them; I would be a living sitcom for their viewing pleasure. So I gave in; at least I would be in control this time. There would be no more hook-ups, set-ups, or blind dates for this pathetic dating game loser. I'll get my own crappy dates, thank you very much.

I went through the obligatory and humiliating shame of creating a dating service video. I don't recommend this process to anyone. Okay, we are going to put this video camera on you, and in a five minute segment you need to be intriguing, charming, witty, sexy, and intelligent all at the same time. And for God's sake, don't look like a deer caught in the headlights.

I did one better, and I managed to look like a deer with its eyes glued shut. For some reason, I couldn't manage to keep my eyes open while I was talking. Was it a nervous response or a mild seizure? I'll never know. What I do know is that men can indeed find a closed eyed babbling woman attractive. I received several invitations for dates, but I thought that the men were either too old, too divorced, or too "not what I was looking for."

I decided that I preferred to do the inviting, so I took the plunge and invited three potential suitors on a date. I found one particular suitor quite intriguing. He seemed intelligent, and I thought that he just might have that oh-so-attractive Renaissance man potential. And besides, his video was just as quirky as mine. While I was struggling to keep my eyes open, this guy was so animated and engaged in his own thoughts that he could not keep his hands from flailing as he talked.

In addition, we both answered the Godforsaken standard dating service questions in the same way. Describe your perfect date. Do you fall in love easily? How would friends describe you? Tell us about your greatest achievement. I always thought that there were a few questions that were missing in the interview: Tell us how you have come to a point in your life in which you feel that it is necessary to answer inane questions and degrade yourself in front of a video camera just so that you can get a date. Would your friends and neighbors describe you as pathetic? Have you always been a loser in the dating scene? Ugh, it was all so silly, contrived, and demeaning, but we had both endured it, and it seemed as if we just might be sharing the same brain. This guy definitely had potential.

After a few days of waiting, my potential Renaissance man called and left a message on my answering machine. Such excitement and such terror I have never felt. My first instinct was to jump up and down and scream in fits of glee, but that thought was quickly tempered by the realization that I suddenly had an acute and overwhelming urge to heave the contents of my stomach. My partially digested dinner was now churning with an unbridled ferocity, and I decided that it would be wise to hold my one-woman celebratory party in the bathroom.

After gathering enough courage to go onto the dating service battlefield, I returned his call the following day, and we chatted for a good hour. Hmm, he still seemed intelligent, and we seemed to have a great deal in common, so we agreed to meet on the third of July for dinner and fireworks by the lakefront, a popular Milwaukee tradition. Now the sheer terror really washed over me. Good grief, I'm going on a date with a guy I have never met. What if I end up as the cover story in tomorrow's paper? I could just see the headline screaming, "Stupid Woman Murdered after Picking Bad Seed for Date!"

I had yet to tell my family that I had joined the dating service, so I told a friend about the date, and I told her that if I turned up missing, she would be responsible for relaying all of the facts to the police and placing my photograph on the sides of milk cartons. I also decided that it would be wise to buy some pepper spray. I reasoned that if the bad seed made a lecherous advance or tried to use a chainsaw on me, I would be more than prepared. My flair for the dramatic was in high gear, and I was prepared for all of the possible scenarios, as

I was about to embark on my first venture into the wild world of the dating service.

The day of our first date finally arrived, and my anxiety had reached a fevered pitch. I began the day by taking the kind of shower that people normally reserve for big job interviews and yearly physical exams. I had always believed that cleanliness was next to godliness, and after thirty minutes in the bathtub, I was clean and shiny enough to be canonized.

My body was perfectly clean, and it was now my mouth's turn to feel the wrath of first date preparations. Since good breath is always critical on a first date, I brushed and flossed my teeth with such zeal that my gums were slightly shredded. The resulting sting and pain of the alcohol laden mouthwash nearly brought tears to my eyes. I was beginning to remember why I detested dating. The ritualistic behavior surrounding a first date was not only ridiculous, it was painful. The concept of an arranged marriage began to seem slightly appealing.

My next challenge was to begin the quest for the perfect outfit. I had a closet full of clothing, but I suddenly had nothing to wear. I changed my clothing countless times, and before long, my entire wardrobe was crumpled into small heaps on the bathroom floor. I was clean enough to meet even the strictest standards of Leviticus, but I had nothing to cover my squeaky clean flesh. And since nudity was not an option on the first date, I finally settled on a stylish but casual combination of jeans and a forest green blouse. I was no centerfold, but I was pleasantly pleased with my appearance.

I was finally ready to embark on my evening's adventure, so I did a final butt check in the mirror, checked my hair from every possible angle, adjusted my bra one final time, grabbed my pepper spray, and made my way to the garage. There was no turning back now. I was now fully prepared to meet my fate or my destiny.

I had to drive to downtown Milwaukee, which was a fairly daunting task for me. I was born and raised in the suburbs, and the concept of parallel parking and densely populated areas naturally overwhelmed me. I was the ultimate suburban white girl who felt compelled to pack and prepare for any venture into the downtown area. I filled the car's gas tank, locked myself in the car, and placed my map, pepper spray, and bottled water strategically on the passenger's seat. I could navigate, defend, and hydrate myself within seconds if necessary. This fifteen-minute trip to the city was fraught with danger, but I was willing to journey into the belly of the beastly city for a chance to meet the Renaissance man. I was on a quest for love, and I was packed and prepared for the journey.

Naturally, when I arrived downtown, parking and navigating were indeed issues. I wasn't sure where I was going, and I didn't know where to park. Once I stumbled upon the restaurant, I must have circled around it five times in an attempt to find a parking spot. On my fifth swing around the block, I saw the Renaissance man standing on the corner, and I secretly prayed that he had not witnessed my feeble attempt at navigating the city. Unfortunately, I found out several months later that he had indeed seen me circling aimlessly, but he was kind enough not to mention my navigational ineptness on our first date.

Our first date went very well. We had dinner in a charmingly homey pub along the Milwaukee River, and I made sure that I ate almost everything on my plate. I love food, and since I believe that eating is one of life's greatest pleasures, I wanted this guy to know that I was no dainty salad-eating girl. He would either have to accept me as is or return me to the dating service. It would be as simple as returning a pair of shoes. She doesn't fit; I need a different size.

Our conversations were steady and interesting throughout the entire dinner. We discussed our families, our jobs, our interests, and we even touched briefly upon our relationship history. It was a potentially dangerous topic, and I suddenly wished that I had more of a past. I felt like Mother Theresa when I was able to summarize my love history in one minute and thirty seconds. But I was thrilled when Doug's history only took about two minutes and thirty seconds. Doug had dated significantly more than I, and his relationship history did take a full minute longer to relate, but we did discover that serious relationships and love had been elusive for both of us.

Our steady stream of conversation continued as we moved to the lakefront to watch the fireworks. We seemed to have so much in common, and I couldn't help thinking that he felt like a comfortable old friend. It was great to watch the fireworks with him, and I was mesmerized by the way the colors in the sky lit up his face as he talked. I was slowly letting my guard down, and I was happy to discover that I was completely content standing next to this stranger. His words swirled in my mind, and I realized that the Renaissance man was living up to all of my expectations. On that warm July evening, I knew that at the very least I had a new friend.

Among our many similarities, we shared a penchant for protecting ourselves. I discovered that he was also carrying a personal safety item: a small alarm that wailed like a banshee at the push of a button. I told him that I had pepper spray, and we laughed at the thought that the common criminal on the streets of Milwaukee didn't stand a chance against us. In reality, I mentioned the spray to let him know that I was an armed woman and that I wasn't afraid to use force on him. But Doug was a perfect gentleman, and there would be no need for pepper spray. We both agreed that we had had a very pleasant evening, and we decided that we definitely wanted to go out on another date.

As we said our goodbyes in my car, Doug patted me on the shoulder, and I felt obliged to give him a signal to let him know that he had potential for joining the Dana club. My mind raced as I tried to decide what gesture would be appropriately charming and endearing. I made a quick decision to lightly pat his knee, and at the exact moment in which my hand made contact with his pants, I lamented my choice. There was a smorgasbord of body parts that I could have chosen, but for some reason, I chose the always unattractive and knobby knee. It is a body part that no one really likes or finds attractive, but I was drawn to his knee as if it were magnetized. I was certain that I had blown everything with my stupid knee pat. For God's sake, who pats a guy's knee? Well, I know who. People who have to join dating services, that's who. But hey, I did get a second date, so maybe there is something to the under recognized and under appreciated allure of the knobby knee pat.

Doug and I went to a nature center for our second date, and the nervousness that surrounded me on our first date continued to be a problem. I was more than capable of maintaining and enjoying our conversations, but I had to constantly focus on quelling the overwhelming nausea that enveloped me whenever I was in his presence. Did I really like him, or did I have intestinal parasites? The distinction between the sensations of love and parasites can be very confusing to the untrained heart and stomach.

My nausea was also heightened because I was extremely self-conscious about a blemish that had decided to take up residence on my face just a few days prior to our date. In an attempt to look my best, I had decided to put a huge glob of acne medication on the offending beast and cover it with a Band-Aid the evening before our date. Unfortunately, the next morning when I attempted to remove the Band-Aid, some of the skin came off, and I was left with a red Band-Aid silhouette. So in addition to the original pulsating pimple, I now had a Band-Aid injury to highlight it. I did my best to rest my face on my hand in an attempt to cover the carnage. I even thought that the hand on the face trick might even make me look charmingly coy, but I eventually decided that I should just let my face be seen—blemish and all.

In spite of the face disaster, Doug invited me on a third date. This time we went to the art museum in Chicago, and it was during this trip that he revealed to me for the first time that he had cystic fibrosis. I knew very little about the disease, but I did know that it was disease that could kill its victims at a very young age.

I had seen the movie *Alex: The Life of a Child* when I was about eighteen, and I vividly remembered the horrible cough and the death of the young girl. For some odd reason, I also remembered the scene in which the girl is dying and her last wish is to have a sip of root beer. Her father leaves her side to go to the grocery store, and he is delayed by a woman who will not stop talking at the cash register. I remembered thinking that when I started to do my own grocery shopping, I would never chat with a cashier for very long. My eighteen-year-old mind reasoned that I could never know if there was someone behind me who was attempting to purchase someone's last wish.

So now I was sitting next to a grown man who had this disease, and I immediately wondered why he was still alive. I reasoned that I just didn't know anything about the disease, and I assumed that he must just have a "touch" of CF. Being naïve was pleasant and comforting, but the comfort of my ignorance would be very short-lived.

After returning from Chicago, I was plagued by a desire to learn more about this disease. I knew that I liked this guy, and I felt certain that the relationship had potential. He seemed to embody everything for which I was searching. But I was so overwhelmed by a sense of melancholy that he might be very sick, and I was also overwhelmed by a sense of selfishness. I knew that this disease was going to complicate and ruin everything in our new relationship. But before I buried this guy and the relationship, I also knew that I needed to understand more about the disease.

I went to the library, and I checked out two books. When I returned home, I placed them on my coffee table and just stared at them for several hours. I was scared to death to open them; I was afraid of the ugly reality that they might reveal. There were two loaded guns on my coffee table, and I was playing Russian Roulette with them. Were the books dangerously loaded, or were they harmless?

I eventually read both of the books, and there were words and sentences that resonated in my overwhelmed and confused mind. The word fatal leapt from the pages over and over and danced endlessly in my brain. I found myself re-reading a sentence that stated that most people with CF are dead by the age of thirty. Dead by the age of thirty? Doug was twenty-nine years old, so I reasoned that he was living on borrowed time, as was this new relationship.

I also discovered among the pages of the books that 98 percent of all males with CF are sterile. If I were to pursue a relationship with this man, any hope of having children was quickly dashed. I was sitting in my apartment feeling empty and sorry for myself, but what I didn't realize was that I was a very lucky woman who was about to embrace the uncertainty of life and embark on the greatest and most rewarding journey of her life.

Love and a cough cannot be hid.
—George Herbert

Embracing Uncertainty

I would love to tell you that I didn't give Doug's illness a second thought and that I just jumped at the chance to begin a relationship with him. I did continue to see him, but I was initially plagued by constant fear and uncertainty. Quite honestly, I wasn't sure if I had the emotional fortitude to deal with the unpleasant possibilities of his disease. I wanted a nice and simple life, and I wanted a healthy boyfriend.

As time passed, and my fondness grew for him, my focus gradually drifted away from his health. I ultimately decided that Doug deserved to be loved just as much as anyone else did, and if I were to end the relationship solely based on his illness, then I would be a shallow and heartless woman. Fortunately for both of us, my ego just could not handle the prospect of being either shallow or heartless. I had always tried to live my life according to the Golden Rule, and this was not the time to change that philosophy. Doug needed me just as much as I needed him.

Our relationship progressed just as any other normal relationship would; we were smitten and stupid. We did all of the normal things that couples do as they progress through the relationship building process: we talked and laughed endlessly as we went to restaurants, plays, movies, and concerts. We basked in the glow of the wonderful and joyous simplicity of just sitting at home and watching TV with someone with whom you are falling in love. Mundane tasks suddenly became exciting, and the harsh world seemed to soften in the shadow of our new relationship. Oh, what a wondrous and glorious process falling in love is. But the process is not quite so simple and glorious when cystic fibrosis is a part of the picture.

In January of 1995, I experienced my first dose of CF reality. Doug had been on IV antibiotics for a lung infection when he suddenly began to cough up blood. He was alone in his apartment, and he had just gone to bed when he heard a gurgling sound in his lungs. Having lived with hemoptysis (coughing up blood) for years, Doug knew immediately what the gurgle would inevitably bring. Indeed, the gurgle led to a cough which then led to a seemingly endless flow of bright red blood.

He sat alone in his apartment for three hours coughing up blood. In an attempt to calm himself, he called his good friend in North Carolina who also happened to be a doctor. Through tears, he asked her how in the world he could ask me to live with this. How fair was it to ask a young and healthy woman to accept the burden of his illness? She encouraged him to calm down and call an ambulance immediately. Emotionally charged philosophical banter would have to wait; he needed medical care. He obliged and anxiously awaited the arrival of the ambulance.

While waiting, he went to the window and stared out at the city. He lived on the eighth floor of a high-rise apartment building in downtown Milwaukee, and he had a spectacular view of the heart of the city. Despite the fact that it was late, the city was still vibrantly full of life. People bustled on the streets, cars passed by, and the city lights twinkled brightly. As he looked down, he marveled at the world from which he felt completely removed.

Illness provides unrelenting and unpredictable uncertainty, but it does manage to be consistently predictable in the fact that it isolates its victims, and that reality is never clearer than in the midst of fear and suffering. Doug's health and life were uncertain, but on that night, he was certain of the fact that there was a girl he loved, and there was a girl who was going to be hurt by his love.

The following day, Doug called me at work at the end of the day. He told me about his night, and he asked if he could come and stay with me for a few days. My mind raced as I tried to comprehend the magnitude of coughing up blood. The fears that I had managed to stifle for the past few months rose up again and began to suffocate me. Was I really strong enough for this? Why did such a great guy have to deal with this? Why did I have to deal with this? I pushed these thoughts aside and quickly rushed downtown to rescue him.

He was waiting in the lobby of his apartment, and I was never so happy to see him. He looked so tired and weary, but his face lit up at the very sight of me. I hugged him, and I remember feeling an overwhelming sense of being complete in his presence. I melted into him, and I knew at that moment that I truly loved him and that I could, without question, face the uncertainty of his disease. I knew that I had been blessed with a relationship that some people only dream of, and I knew that I would be eternally grateful no matter how long it was destined to last.

When we got into the car, he began to share his ordeal with me. Doug was never one to lament his reality, but on this day, he opened his soul and bared all of his pain and fear. Our relationship immediately deepened as he slowly and methodically began to relay the events of the previous evening, his brief hospital stay, and his morning.

After being released from the hospital, he took a taxi back to his apartment, and as the taxi was pulling away, he remembered that he needed to go to the grocery store. But he was too tired and hungry for grocery shopping, so he decided that would eat whatever he could find, take a shower, and then go for groceries. When he hopped in the shower, he quickly realized that the plumbing in the old cream city brick building had failed him again, and he was destined to struggle through yet another cold shower.

As he dressed after his shower, he noticed a photograph of himself as a child on the floor of his closet. He picked up the black and white photograph and began to examine and dissect the happiness in the face of the child. The child wore a face of ignorance and bliss: an emotion and state to which this grown man could no longer relate. Doug grieved for the child he once was, for the child who stared back at him could not have known how difficult life would eventually become. The innocence of childhood had mercifully sheltered him from the full reality of his illness, and he once again longed for the comfort and shelter of that innocence.

His introspective mood continued as he made his way to the grocery store. As he was walking around the store, he watched the other people moving aimlessly down the aisles, and he marveled at the routine nature and necessity of grocery shopping. And then he began to silently wonder what secret heartache each person held inside. As human beings, we are the walking wounded. Each person has had his or her share of heartache and misfortune, but life moves on no matter what it hands us. It demands that we move on, so we don our masks of happiness, and we move through our lives carrying the constant burden of something lost or unattained.

As I listened to his story, my heart ached for him. However, I could not help wondering why he didn't call me. I was angry that he had subjected himself to facing this ordeal alone. I asked him why he didn't call, and he told me that he didn't want to wake me; he didn't want me to worry or be scared. I promptly told him that I was now a part of his life and that if he wanted me to continue being a part of his life, he needed to be open with me and rely on me. I told him that I would never leave him because of his disease. I could handle his illness, but I could not handle being shut out emotionally.

Doug had always handled his illness on his own, and it was initially difficult for him to relinquish some of that control. It took time and several reminders, but he eventually allowed me to shoulder some of the burden. The physical battle would forever be on his shoulders, but he could now allow someone else to share part of the emotional load. For the first time in his life, he began to see a future, and he realized fully and completely that a woman could see past his illness and love him for who he was. It was on that day that Doug told me that he loved me for the first time. I echoed his sentiments, and we reveled in the boundless possibilities of our future.

More marriages might survive if the partners realized that sometimes the better comes after the worse.

—Doug Larson

He is Mine Today

Doug proposed to me on March 17, 1995. We had spent the day together, and as evening approached, a friend of mine came over to help me prepare for a bridal shower that I was hosting the following day. While we were in the kitchen, Doug stayed in the family room watching basketball. He seemed jittery, and I was befuddled as to why he was watching sports on TV. After all, this was my Renaissance man, and he never watched sports.

From time to time, I would glance over at him, and I would notice that he didn't really seem to be watching the game. I did, however, notice that his legs were constantly bouncing, and he would throw a nervous glance in my direction at regular intervals. I was confused by his behavior, and I silently wondered if I had fallen in love with a man who had a personality disorder.

After we had finished cooking, my friend left, and Doug became even more anxious. I paid little attention to his bizarre behavior because I was focused on cleaning the kitchen. In addition to my many neuroses, I have a cleaning neurosis. I absolutely love to clean, and I could not rest until that darn kitchen was shining again. Besides, I reasoned, I was hosting a party tomorrow, and I wanted the apartment to look as fine as a tiny one bedroom apartment could possibly look. Doug continued to beg me to stop, but I protested that I could not focus on anything until I had finished the cleaning.

When I finally had the kitchen in pristine condition, I walked over to the couch and asked him what in the world had gotten into him. His face lit up, and he grinned like a cat that had just feasted on a family of mice. He told me that he had something for me, and he handed me a 3x5 note card. It contained a clue that I had to solve, and when I had solved it, it would lead me to another card.

It took me a while to complete the scavenger hunt, but at the end, there was a card with a drawing of a diamond ring. I turned to see him standing beside me with a jewelry box. He opened it slowly, and I gazed upon a golden engagement ring. I looked into his eyes, and I saw such a look of excitement and anticipation that it overwhelmed me. The happiness in his eyes was radiant, and I marveled at how the sadness that I had seen in his eyes just a few months earlier now seemed so distant.

My mind also drifted back to the childhood photo that he had described to me at that same time. I imagined that the face I now gazed upon must surely resemble the look of happiness that he wore as a child. His childhood innocence was forever gone, but the happiness had returned. He proposed, and I accepted. Cystic fibrosis would not claim this moment; it was ours, and nothing could take it from us.

We began the process of planning our wedding, and I must admit that the process was a bit foreign to me. I was not your typical girl. I had never pictured myself in a wedding dress, and I had certainly never spent any time planning my dream wedding.

I decided to buy some bridal magazines, and as I glanced through the glossy pages, I was quickly repulsed by the thought of wearing a wedding dress. I hated dresses with an intensity not to be rivaled. I continued to thumb through the pages of these magazines for days, and I mused at the frilly dresses, the flowers, the cakes, and the countless sex articles.

Oh dear, the sex articles seemed to be more abundant than anything else in the magazine: "How to Please Your Man," "Real Guys Confess Their Wedding Fantasies," and "How to Turn on Your Groom." I felt so overwhelmed. I had to wear a dress and provide some earth shattering wedding night fantasy all in the same day? Was there no end to this wedding insanity? All of this was so "girly," and "girly" was about the last adjective that could ever describe me. I decided to forego the advice from the magazines and just focus on creating a ceremony that would reflect our personalities.

We quickly picked a cake, a reception hall, music, our wedding rings; dresses for the bridesmaids, tuxedos, and flowers. What else was there? Oh yes, that damn dress. I tried on a few dresses, but each time I looked in the mirror, I almost had a convulsion. I just didn't look right in a dress. Of course, as my mother had always pointed out, I did have a tendency to slump over whenever a dress came near my body. My spine did have a tendency to give way in a dress' presence, but I wasn't sure how to overcome this problem.

My second problem was that virtually every dress available had ten pounds of lace and a big bow on the backside. I didn't think that I had a big butt, but I did know that it was always good practice to avoid drawing attention to an area that has such a profound potential for being problematic. Besides, I had read so many of the sex articles in the bridal magazines that I had become paranoid, and the thought of slapping a bow on my butt and parading around with it terrified me. I just knew that people would think that I was giving my ass to Doug as a wedding gift. It just seemed tasteless, sleazy, and inappropriate.

I can't remember whose idea it was, but we somehow stumbled upon the idea of wearing my mother's wedding dress. I tried it on, and my spine stayed amazingly upright. I thought that the top bared just a bit too much flesh, and I accused my mother of being a harlot on her wedding day. Luckily, Doug's mother had worked at a clothing store, and there was a wonderful seamstress who was able to make a Bolero style jacket to cover my flesh. It was a perfect solution, and I was proud and honored to wear the same dress that my mother had worn on her wedding day.

By the time we had finished choosing everything for the wedding, we had grown weary of the whole process, and we just wanted to get married. I couldn't wait to marry him, but I was really quite nervous about the ceremony. I have never liked being the center of attention, and the thought of having seventy-five pairs of eyes boring into my skull did not thrill me.

Doug, however, reveled in the limelight, and he was anxiously looking forward to having his rock star moment. What I did not know at the time, however, was that Doug was struggling with his own wedding issues. He was not concerned about tuxedos, dresses, butt bows, or the watchful eyes of wedding guests. He was concerned about trying to stay alive for me. Before our wedding ceremony, he had asked God to give me at least five years with him.

The day of our wedding finally arrived. It was a cool, cloudy, and blustery fall day. I was excited and ridiculously nervous. I had no reservations about marrying Doug, but I had serious reservations about parading down an aisle in a dress. Would my spine hold up? Would I be able to keep my breakfast down? I was normally so philosophical at moments like these, but my thoughts had been reduced to a primal survival level. Finally, my moment of truth had come, and I was ready to proceed down the aisle flanked by my parents.

I looked to my left and to my right, and I saw that I was surrounded by the most important people in my life. I was overwhelmed by the fact that these people were gathered here in our name, and I was immediately stuck by the fact that this exact collection of people would never be gathered again. I also wondered if I should greet people as I strolled down the aisle. It seemed so rude to just pass by without saying hello. Damn those bridal magazines—not one of them had mentioned appropriate wedding-march etiquette.

So as I began to stroll down the aisle, I decided to greet people as if I were the Queen of England on a publicity tour. People giggled as I greeted them, and I was thrilled with my decision to meet and greet as I strode down the aisle. But then I looked straight ahead, and I saw Doug. Instantaneously, all of the other people and all of my extemporaneous thoughts evaporated, and it was just the two of us. I looked into his eyes, and I was overcome by the profundity of the experience. I was pledging my love to this one person; I was about to commit every part of my being to this man. Looking back, his disease was never further from my mind than at that particular moment.

We proceeded through the ceremony, and we finally reached the part of the ceremony in which we were to exchange our vows. As I turned toward Doug and looked into his eyes, I saw the haziness of his tears, and I knew that we were in serious trouble. He struggled through his vows, and I struggled desperately to maintain my composure. I knew that if I succumbed to the emotions that I was feeling, I would end up on the floor as a weeping mass of off-white satin.

It was now my turn. I repeated my vows, and again, it was as if no one else was in the church. I managed to get through everything until I had to repeat the line, "In sickness and health." I immediately thought of the implications of the line, and I wondered how many people have stumbled through those words without contemplating their true meaning. The words overwhelmed me, and the joy of the day was momentarily replaced by tremendous sadness.

I knew that sickness would be an integral part of our marriage, and I suddenly ached for our future. But as I looked into Doug's eyes, I was filled with an intense resolve to maintain my hold on this moment. This was our moment, and cystic fibrosis would not steal it. So I said my vows, and I silently cursed the disease that had dared to intrude upon our day.

We completed the ceremony and retreated back down the aisle as husband and wife to the tune of Beethoven's "Ode to Joy." When we exited the church, we stopped in the vestibule and allowed ourselves to succumb completely to the emotion of the day. We were alone and engulfed in an odd combination of pure joy and profound sadness. We loved one another completely, and this was the best day of our lives. But our hearts ached for our uncertain future. I wanted to cling to the moment and hold Doug forever in an attempt to protect him from the ugliness of his disease. If we could just stay in the moment, time could not move forward, and cystic fibrosis could not take him from me. But I ultimately knew that we had to move forward. I acknowledged the fact that cystic fibrosis had laid its claim upon my husband, and I also acknowledged the fact that I would not relinquish him without a tremendous fight. And on our wedding day, I spoke to the invisible intruder, "He is mine today, and there is no time for sadness or fear. You are not welcome here."

Fear knocked on the door. Faith answered. No one was there.

—Anonymous

The Naughty Child in the Corner

Our marriage began like any other marriage. We were a young couple with a new apartment and a room full of wedding gifts. Youth and wedding gifts are always the perfect recipe for bliss or disaster. But our life was good and blissful, and we felt like our future was full of nothing but promise.

I was still teaching at the same suburban high school, and Doug was working on his doctoral dissertation while teaching philosophy at Marquette University. We worked during the week, grumbled about the occasional ineptness of our students, and had fun on the weekends. We loved eating out, going to Bed and Breakfasts, and we relished any opportunity to see a movie. Doug had a penchant for foreign movies or anything that didn't make sense, and I was smitten by anything that could be dumped into the category of romantic comedy or drama. After getting married, I had finally achieved that stereotypical romantic girl quality that I had lacked for so many years.

Cystic fibrosis rarely intruded during the early years of our marriage, but its presence was a constant fixture in our lives. The disease was like a third person, and I likened it to an extremely naughty and out of control child who was always sitting the in the corner of the room for a time out. We knew that we could usually keep a reign on the beast if he stayed in the corner, but we just never knew when he would stand up, rumble out of the corner, and wreak havoc on our lives.

Despite the sometimes-quiet CF periods, Doug's daily medical routine was a constant fixture that was time intensive and involved. Each morning, he would get up, take a handful of pills, and nebulize a dose of Albuterol and Pulmozyme (a mucous thinner). He would then perform chest physiotherapy (CPT). Since sticky and copious amounts of mucous fills the lungs of individuals with cystic fibrosis, it is essential to use some form of daily therapy to help keep the lungs as clear as possible. Doug's method of attack was the Flutter. The Flutter is a device that looks like a tiny peace pipe, but there is a ball inside of the pipe that causes a vibration in the lungs when air is forced into it. The idea behind the Flutter is to cause vibrations that will aid in breaking the mucous loose so that it is more easily coughed up and out of the lungs.

Following his chest therapy, Doug would then inhale an antibiotic via his nebulizer. He would have to alternate his antibiotics every two to four weeks in an attempt to reduce the resistance of the bacteria that colonized his lungs. This entire process would take about two hours each morning, and he then had to repeat the same routine every evening. The entire process was a tedious nuisance, and we hated the countless hours that it consumed over time. But the routine was a necessary evil, and we knew that it kept him alive and relatively healthy.

Cystic fibrosis not only wreaks its havoc on the lungs, but it also affects the digestive system. Fortunately, Doug's GI system has never been severely affected by the disease. However, like many other CF patients, Doug has to take pancreatic enzymes to help him digest his food. Doctors refer to this problem as malabsorption, and it can lead to intestinal blockages, malnourishment, poor weight gain, and poor health.

In addition to the problem of malabsorption, the tremendous energy that is consumed by breathing requires that most patients eat a tremendous number of calories. When I married Doug, he weighed 119 pounds soaking wet. But after a year or so of marriage, his weight ballooned to a very healthy 140 pounds. I often joked that there was nothing like the cooking of a good woman. I couldn't believe that the girl who once gave little thought or attention to men and marriage was now making marital cooking jokes. It was a wonder that I wasn't swapping recipes and coupons with the ladies in the neighborhood. Dear Lord, I had become domestic, and I seemed to be enjoying it. But no matter what, I was not going to quilt or cross-stitch. There was still a level of domesticity that I was unwilling to accept.

I have always marveled at Doug's ability to stay focused and regimented with his health, and I can honestly say that I rarely heard him complain about his daily treatments or therapies. He was so focused on maintaining his health that absolutely nothing could break his determination and drive. I would whine about flossing my teeth every night, so I can hardly imagine what sort of annoying creature I would have been if I had been the one with the disease.

Doug had been a poster child for a local cystic fibrosis chapter in the Chicago area when he was nine years of age, and his desire to maintain his poster child stature continued into adulthood: he saw his doctor without fail, washed his hands regularly, did all of his treatments daily, took his meds, and exercised. But despite his fastidious care, he would still have exacerbations that would require IV antibiotics once or twice a year.

He could always tell that he was getting sick because his cough would increase, his sputum would thicken or change colors, and he would feel lethargic. I could sometimes tell that Doug was getting sick before he could because I would notice what I called his "sick face." His face would take on an ashen pallor, and I would say, "You have your sick face. How are you feeling?" My emotions hung on the color of his face, the frequency and depth of every cough, and his energy level. I, like Doug, did my best to control his health, but we ultimately knew that despite our very best efforts, the disease had a mind of its own.

I can still remember the first time that he had to have IV antibiotics after we were married. There was a home health care company that was going to come to our apartment, provide the IV drugs, and place his PICC line. The nurse showed up with a nurse-in-training, and after filling out a mountain of paperwork, they began the process of placing his line. When the nurse pulled out the needle that would provide the lead for his IV line, I did my best to not contort my face in anguish. In my medically untrained mind, this needle would have been better suited for a horse.

Unfortunately, Doug had the opportunity to experience the pure joy of this horse needle several times, as the nurse couldn't seem to position it properly into the vein. I remembered thinking that the whole process reminded me of a game of "pin the tail on the donkey" at a child's birthday party. Hey, it's a party. Just blindfold his wife, hand her the needle, and let her take a stab at it. We only needed paper party hats, a cake, and some fruit punch to complete the picture.

When the nurse finally managed to strike gold, she was a little slow in feeding the line, and I was appalled to see my husband's blood spewing from the lead. Fortunately, Doug was looking away, but after a short time he stated that his arm felt fairly wet. "Is that blood that I'm feeling?" The nurse responded by telling him that it was just a little bit. My mind was reeling, and my sarcastic thoughts were pleading for freedom: Hello? A little bit? If I were to spill a gallon of milk on your head, would you believe me if I told you that it was just a little bit? Good grief, woman.

Doug eventually turned his head, looked down at what now looked like the scene of an autopsy, and almost passed out. The student nurse looked as white as Doug, and she was momentarily rendered useless. So I, the Spanish teacher, helped the other nurse get Doug over to the couch before he passed out. I was stunned when the nurse asked him if he normally had fainting issues. Hey lady, who doesn't have fainting issues when they have lost a third of their blood supply? My virgin introduction to home IV's was overwhelming, and I was astonished by the fact that an outpatient surgery had just occurred on my dining room table.

We did have the home care company place his PICC lines a few more times, but every experience was bad, and Doug's doctor eventually decided to have the lines placed in a hospital setting.

Hospital or living room—is there really any difference? Yes, that sentence is just laced with the sarcasm of an overprotective wife.

Despite the occasional IV's and hemoptysis, Doug's health remained relatively stable for the first five or six years of our marriage. But around 2000, he slowly began to show signs of deterioration. In August of 2000, he was hospitalized with necrotizing pneumonia, and he then suffered another round of pneumonia early in 2001. He bounced back each time, but we were becoming increasingly afraid of just how much bounce he had left in those old lungs.

Unfortunately, 2002 didn't provide much of a respite for Doug either. He started to have more shortness of breath, and he began using oxygen for sleeping and exercising. The day that the oxygen compressor was brought into our home was a very difficult day. For the first time, we had machinery that confirmed his decline. We logically and rationally knew that he was declining, but this machine screamed the reality loudly and clearly.

But not to be outdone by his disease, Doug increased his level of activity by walking on the treadmill and lifting weights. We rationalized that although we could not reverse the damage that was already done to his lungs, we could at least do our best to keep it at bay for as long as possible. Doug exercised, and I cooked healthy meals, researched the disease endlessly online, and started him on a vitamin regimen. But our attempts to soothe and stop the proverbial naughty child would be in vain. The child had finally risen with a vengeance from his corner, and he would not be subdued this time. His full ugliness was unleashed, and it quickly became evident that he would never return to his corner.

On November 7, 2002, Doug was listed for a bilateral lung transplant at University Hospital and Clinics in Madison, Wisconsin. Even then, we comforted ourselves by believing that we could get him healthy enough to become inactive on the list. But again, the disease would not relent. In January of 2003, Doug needed IV antibiotics again after coughing up blood. His x-rays showed another lung infection, and he spent three days in the hospital. After he was released, he began to feel better and stronger than he had in a while, and we began to hope again.

But just as hope will float, it will also sink. In February, I managed to contract a horrible case of the flu, and despite our best precautions, Doug also managed to get sick. He ended up in the hospital, and his lung function dipped to a paltry 16 percent. He also began to use oxygen twenty-four hours a day, and for the first time, I wondered if he could stay healthy long enough to survive the average two year wait for a transplant.

His doctor confirmed my worst fears when she gently encouraged us to investigate other hospitals in search of a shorter waiting list. My mind raced as I struggled to comprehend the meaning of the words that fell like daggers from her mouth. My heart sank, and the loud and constant ticking of the clock of my husband's life began to fill the room. I silently panicked as I began to understand the fact that my husband was slipping through my fingers, and I was completely powerless to stop it.

I quickly began the process of researching other hospitals and exploring all of our options. I would spend twelve or thirteen hours with Doug at the hospital, and I would then come home and do research online. I was always amazed by the deafening silence and emptiness that pervaded our condo each night as I struggled to focus on the words and statistics on the computer screen. I had never felt more alone and frightened in my life.

But I was on a mission, and so I took copious notes, and I was heartened to find that there were other hospitals that seemed to have shorter waiting lists. But these hospitals were far away, and some of them were not covered by our insurance company. I agonized day and night about how we would finance everything, what we would do if we had to move to a different state, and what I would do about my job if we had to move.

I had always prided myself in my ability to problem solve, but my fear and desperation were beginning to cloud my ability to focus and remain rational. I just knew that there had to be a solution; there had to be a way to keep him alive. But I would soon discover that all of my worrying and anguish would be for naught.

On March 31, 2003, after only five months on the transplant list, Doug received a call from his transplant coordinator after just stepping out of the shower. With shaving cream still dripping from his face, he heard the words, "Doug, how would you like a new pair of lungs today?"

No matter how dull, or how mean, or how wise a man is, he feels that happiness is his indisputable right.

—Helen Keller

Coping

Our personal struggle with cystic fibrosis has been the greatest challenge of our lives, and it has taken a great deal of effort and soul searching to come to terms with it. My husband and I cannot and could not control cystic fibrosis. We did everything in our power to control and tame it, but despite our best efforts, it ultimately destroyed his lungs.

What cystic fibrosis did not destroy was our relationship and our resolve to battle it to the end. We could not control its path, but we could control how we chose to respond to it. We chose hope, and though there were days when that hope seemed to fade to a flicker, it was never extinguished.

Over the years, we learned that coping with an illness is a daily struggle and endeavor that involves relinquishing the illusion that we are in control, releasing the notion that life is supposed to be fair, trusting in God and others, and laughing in the face of the disease that we loathe.

Human beings naturally crave control. But let's look at the irony here. First, we are thrown unwittingly into a world that is inherently chaotic and out of control. And unlike any other species, we are given the intellectual power to comprehend and live under the illusion that we can control the chaos. I truly think that this might be one of God's best jokes. I imagine God saying, "Here is the greatest gift that you will ever receive: it is your life. Do your best to understand it, treasure it, learn from it, and control it, but always remember that I am ultimately in charge here." It's a bit like the old adage, "Men make plans, and God laughs."

But at the same time, I have never believed that we are God's puppets, or that God creates chaos or suffering. I believe that we live in a fallen, unpredictable, and chaotic world in which God still has complete dominion. He rules and watches over us, but He lets us make our own choices. And as a result of this freedom to choose, I know in my heart that as He watches our decisions, He celebrates our humanity and grieves our inhumanity.

Yet despite the fact that we are free to make choices in our lives, there is still so much that we cannot control. There are illnesses and accidents that just happen, and despite their random appearance, I believe that every event, good or bad, happens for a very specific reason. We are put on this earth to learn, and each event in our lives provides an opportunity for growth and understanding. I believe that we are called to embrace and accept that which we cannot control. For it is when we relinquish the need to be in control that we are released from the weight of bearing the world on our shoulders, and we are able to experience true freedom.

As with any serious illness, cystic fibrosis wants to be in control. It demands space and attention in the life of the patient and his or her family. The key is to give it the attention that it demands without allowing it to fill every space and crevice in your soul and in your home.

I am compelled to return to my "naughty-child-in-the-corner" analogy in regard to this illness. We gave cystic fibrosis a corner in our home, and even though it screamed almost daily for more space and attention, we battled the urge to break down and give it what it wanted. It is a cruel disease that robs people of their breath, their hope, their dreams, and their youth. And when you love someone who has this disease, it will do exactly the same thing to you.

CF is a disease that scars the lungs of the patient while it scars the hearts of the family. It leaves no family unscathed by its presence. Parents of children with CF often feel a guilt for which there is often no absolution when they discover that they have given this genetic disease to their child, and healthy siblings struggle to accept the attention that is naturally and necessarily poured upon their "sick" brother or sister. Friends, coworkers, boyfriends, girlfriends, and spouses embrace and love the individual, but these relationships can easily be enveloped and destroyed by the fear and the uncertainty of the disease.

I often longed and ached for days without cystic fibrosis, but I knew that that could never be a reality. The reality is that I hate CF, and I wish that Doug did not have the disease. But at the same time, CF has made Doug the person he is. It has truly shaped his life and personality. He majored in Philosophy because of a deep desire to understand the meaning of life and suffering, and he has an unparalleled zest for life that is due in large part to his illness.

So the man I love so much has been shaped and created by the disease that I hate so much. So do I curse it, or do I thank it? I believe that I must thank it. Doug would not be the man with whom I fell in love, and I would not be the woman I have grown to be. We are better people because of this disease, and we have an appreciation for the beauty and fragility of life. And for that, I will be eternally grateful.

Another key element in coping with a serious illness is to relinquish the notion that life is fair. As human beings we believe that life should and must be fair, and we are quick to shout the battle cry, "This isn't fair," whenever life disappoints us. Accept the fact that life is inherently unfair, and the sting of disappointment and sadness that inevitably follow disillusionment will be eased. If you are a person of faith, remember that we are promised a life full of sadness and pain.

There are twelve million orphans in Africa as a result of the AIDS epidemic, children are neglected and abused, millions of people go to bed hungry, people die unexpectedly in car crashes, the elderly are forgotten and waste away in nursing homes, vibrant people are diagnosed with terminal illnesses, people are shunned or killed because of their beliefs, and children sit alone on school playgrounds and cafeterias because their peers do not accept them.

Let me say it again, life is unfair. There is so much beauty in life, but the reality is that life is hard, and it will challenge and push us to our limits everyday. Accept that fact, and life will be less disappointing, and the moments of beauty and sweetness will be magnified.

My ability to cope with this disease is due in large part to the grace of God. I am simply not strong enough to deal with something as overwhelming as CF without his strength and guidance. My faith has sustained me in a way that nothing else could have. There is an expression that says that "sorrow looks back, worry looks around, and faith looks up." I trust in God, and although there have been several times when I have felt very alone in His presence, I have always known that He is with me and that I am blessed to be a child of God.

But what does it mean to be blessed? I have always struggled when people say that their lives are blessed. It's an expression that we are quick to utter when life is going well. I understand the concept, and I believe whole-heartedly in the beauty of God's blessings. But if someone is struggling or plagued by constant difficulties or sorrow, are we to naturally assume that that person is not blessed and must therefore be cursed?

I believe that we, the happy and the sad, are all blessed. I might even dare to say that those of us who have suffered more than our share of heartache are the truly blessed. There is an inexplicable and profound beauty in suffering, and if we allow ourselves, we can learn so much and grow through our pain. Besides, how much do we really learn from that which is easy? True growth and character usually emerge from that which is dark and difficult.

Beyond God, I have also found great strength through family, friends, and two online support groups. I have always been one to "go it alone." I don't like to depend on other people if I can do something on my own. But human beings are not intended to "go it alone," and we are called to seek the company and support of others.

Cystic fibrosis has forced me to ask for help and depend on others, and I believe that this is just one of the disease's many life lessons that I was destined to learn. I have benefited tremendously from this lesson, and although I still struggle to ask for help, I know that my world is full of family and friends who will be by my side at a moment's notice. My shoulders are simply not big enough for the weight of cystic fibrosis, and I can finally allow myself to be vulnerable and rely on others without feeling weak. The ability to ask for help is a sign of strength, and if I am strong enough to live with this disease, then I am strong enough to ask for help.

In the winter of 2002, I joined a cystic fibrosis online support group. Doug had always isolated himself from other people with CF. He did not want his world to be consumed by the disease, and as medical knowledge increased, he wanted to avoid the issue of bacterial cross-contamination from patient to patient. For years, I had accepted and encouraged his avoidance of other CF patients since this was one of the ways in which we attempted to keep the naughty child in the corner. But as Doug's health deteriorated, I felt a strong need to connect to others who truly understood the challenges of living with the disease.

I decided to join an online support group called Cystic-L. Cystic-L is a group comprised of approximately seven hundred individuals who are CF patients, spouses, parents, friends, and caregivers. I was immediately hooked by the daily emails that were filled with stories that reverberated with a strange combination of disillusionment, fear, happiness, and perseverance. I quickly became engrossed in the joys and sorrows of their lives, and I was thrilled by the opportunity to finally connect with people who truly understood the challenges of cystic fibrosis. I immediately felt less isolated, and I grew as a result of the support and knowledge that these cyber friends unselfishly offered.

It was amazing how easy it was to get caught up in the lives of complete strangers. Shortly after I joined the list, a member of the group had just received her transplant. I was thrilled for her, and I followed the updates on her progress voraciously. I was so anxious to follow her story that I would check for emails at work. I remember going to school one morning and opening my email to find out that she had passed away from complications of her surgery. I found myself seated in front of my computer screen trying to fight back the tears and feeling dazed and outraged by the news.

I hated cystic fibrosis, and I tried desperately to hold on to my emotions. The tears clouded my eyes, but I would not allow them to fall. I had no desire to explain to my coworkers and students that I was crying because a complete stranger had passed away. I had never spoken to or corresponded with this woman, but she shared the common struggle of cystic fibrosis, and that automatically made her a part of my heart. I mourned the senseless loss of life, and a small piece of my heart was chipped away.

There were a few times that I seriously contemplated leaving the list. I often said, "I need this emotional crap like I need a hole in the head." But I stuck with it, and while it has been gut wrenching at times, it has been so therapeutic for me. Doug eventually joined the list after some friendly and forceful cajoling, and we have been regular contributors ever since.

We also joined a group called Second Wind shortly after Doug was placed on the transplant list. It is very similar to Cystic-L, but this group is made up of about three hundred individuals who are waiting for or who have had lung transplants. We are grateful for these two cyber families, and we are honored to call these people our friends.

Finally, there is no greater coping mechanism than laughter. Throughout our years together, Doug and I have always managed to maintain our senses of humor. Laughing in the face of adversity and seeing the humor in the macabre can make even the scariest illness or challenge seem less daunting.

When Doug used to be on home IV's, I would use his IV pole to do pole dances. Now remember, I am a very conservative girl who doesn't even wear dresses. So the concept of me on a pole is just ridiculous and completely out of character. I was always fully clothed, and keeping my balance and avoiding his IV lines always provided a tremendous challenge for me. Also, while attempting to wrap my legs around the pole, I would sing some ridiculous song that I would create off of the top of my head. The sheer ridiculousness of it all and my singing would always make us laugh hysterically.

We also enjoyed making up songs about his medication, bacteria, and sputum. Doug cultured a bacterium called Pseudomonas, and he used an antibiotic called Tobi to suppress it. He also had to take digestive enzymes with every meal, so we created a little jingle to sing whenever the urge overcame us. The words are as follows: "Tobi in the morning, Tobi in the evening, enzymes at supper time, when Pseudomonas is on the rise, Tobi packs a big surprise." Yes, it is bad, and it shows no musical talent at all, but it always made us giggle. Laughing kept us sane, and I am convinced that our ability to see the humor in almost every situation helped to keep Doug happy and relatively healthy.

Despite these coping strategies, Doug and I still succumbed to moments of doubt, self-pity, and angst. There were days that were just overwhelming, and there was nothing better than a good old fashioned tear filled pity party. I believe that this is a healthy and necessary part of coping, but it is important to move forward and avoid the temptation to become immersed in the pain.

Pain and sorrow become familiar companions when living in the shadow of illness, and their familiarity breeds a strange comfort that is sometimes difficult to resist. But tomorrow is a new day that springs forward with hope and the promise of something better. For us, a lung transplant renewed our hope and fulfilled that promise.

Now I know I've got a heart, 'cause it's breaking.
—The Tin Man (The Wizard of Oz)

Spring's Prelude

March 31, 2003 began like any other day in our lives. It was a bright, warm, and sunny Monday morning, and I cringed at the thought of getting up and going to school. There were only two weeks remaining until spring break, and I was counting the remaining days just as fervently as my students.

As I looked out of my bedroom window, I wondered if winter would finally relinquish its icy grip and allow spring to unleash its colorful majesty. I couldn't wait for the spring flowers to make their glorious and triumphant appearance, as their presence always made my mood and spirit soar. Nature's rebirth beckons with the promise of life renewed, but there was no way that I could know just how much promise and life this early spring day held.

It was 11:30 in the morning, and I had already taught three classes and was just putting the finishing touches on my monotonous brown bag lunch when I was told that I had a phone call. There were only ten minutes remaining in my lunch period, and I was annoyed that anyone would dare to interrupt the most sacred time of my day.

I reluctantly walked to the phone, and when I saw my home number on the caller identification screen, my heart skipped a beat. I immediately knew that something was wrong. Doug had just recently been released from the hospital, and he was still recovering at home. My mind raced as I reluctantly put the phone up to my ear. I instinctively knew that I didn't want to hear whatever he had to tell me, but nothing could have prepared me to hear the words, "You're not going to believe this, but UW Madison just called, and they might have some lungs for me."

I could feel the color drain from my face, and I began to slowly step away from the phone in an attempt to distance myself from the news. I was shocked and scared, and my mind struggled futilely to understand the words that I had just heard. "What? Are you ready for this?" I asked. I wanted to go back in time. I wanted to sit at the lunch table again and be oblivious to this news.

There was no joy or excitement; there was only fear. I knew with absolute certainty that I did not want him to take the lungs. I turned to the other teachers in the room and said, "They might have lungs for Doug." People cheered, but their words and faces were unrecognizable to me as I tried desperately to process the thoughts that raced through my mind. I was momentarily lost in my own confusion until I recognized and heard the voice of my friend and colleague of thirteen years, "Dana, this is great news."

"Is it?" I responded.

I walked back to my classroom in a daze. As I gathered my things, the phone rang, and I saw my home number flash on the caller identification screen again. I secretly hoped that Doug was calling to tell me that the lungs were no good. But this phone call would not bring the relief that I sought. His coordinator had called again, and everything was looking like a "go."

I sat down immediately because I was no longer certain that my legs could support me. I had to go home. I had to drive Doug to Madison. I knew this, but my body refused to respond. I felt glued to the chair, and I began to cry. "I don't think I can do this," I said to the two co-workers who were in my classroom. "I know I can't do this," I said to myself.

Just a few weeks earlier, I was desperately trying to find a way to get a transplant for Doug, and now I wanted no part of it. This surgery could kill him, and I was suddenly willing to live with the uncertainty of his CF ridden lungs. Cystic fibrosis offers nothing but uncertainty, but I knew that uncertainty; it was familiar and comfortable. Without the surgery, I knew that he would wake up next to me the following morning; he would still be mine. But this transplant was completely foreign to me, and I knew that it could easily make me a widow by the next sunrise.

I continued to wrestle with my thoughts, and I knew that I would eventually have to get up and face whatever this day and this transplant would bring. I drove home in a fog, and I begged God not to take him as I drove. I was completely unable to see the positive possibilities of this transplant; I could only see the potential for loss and heartache.

When I arrived home, I quickly gathered everything that I thought I might need. I looked around as I packed my bag, and I couldn't help wondering if we would ever be together again in this place that we had called home for five years. There were so many memories enclosed between the walls of our home, and the thought that this might be our final memory in the house almost brought me to my knees. But that thought faded when I realized that we had finally come to the moment that I had dreaded ever since he was placed on the transplant list: the drive to the hospital.

I had pictured this moment in my mind several times, and the thought of it terrified me. What we would say to one another? Would we talk endlessly, or would the ride be fearfully silent? Would we cry, or would we be calm? We were about to embark on our journey, and the answers to the questions that I had feared for five months would soon be revealed.

Madison is about fifty miles from our home, and the drive takes a good solid hour. Oh, how I dreaded this hour. We got on the freeway, and I was amazed by the beauty of day. The sky was clear and brilliantly blue, and the warmth and glow of the sun announced the long awaited prelude to spring. My mind swirled with emotion, but attempting to process any thoughts or ideas quickly became an exercise in futility. I became entranced by the fear and confusion until I suddenly realized that we were driving in complete silence. There was only the rhythmic sound of Doug's portable oxygen machine that dared to break the deafening silence.

I was unsure of everything in my life, but I knew with absolute certainty that we needed to talk. I knew that this could be our last opportunity to talk, but I no longer knew what to say to the man who had been a constant presence in my life for the past nine years. Silence was safe; talking would be painful. But I knew that silence was not an option. We needed to talk, and I wanted no regrets.

We began to talk, and our conversation quickly became an attempt to convince ourselves that this was the right time for a transplant. We knew that Doug's health was failing, but our emotions would not be swayed by logic. No words or rationalizations would ease our minds, and the silence slowly and steadily crept back into the car's interior. Fear and uncertainty would be our traveling companions, and conversation would not come easily on this day.

We drove for several miles until Doug broke the silence again by saying, "I just really want this to work for you." I looked over at him, and I could see the tears gathering in his eyes. I struggled to maintain my composure as the weight and irony of his words fell upon my heart. I was scared for myself, but my thoughts were focused on how much he had endured with this disease, and I was desperate for him to have a successful resolution to his suffering. I wanted the transplant to work for him; he deserved this second chance at life.

We were headed toward personal uncertainty, but we were worried about each other. The meaning of love became apparent to me in a way that it never had before. I was reminded of a line from the second reading at our wedding from 1 Corinthians 13:7 (NLT): Love never gives up, never loses faith, is always hopeful, and endures every circumstance.

I grabbed his hand, and I finally allowed the tears to fall. The emotion was overwhelming, and I did not know how I was going to endure and survive the pain that permeated every part of my being. I needed and craved a respite from the pain, and so I joked that we were going to end up as organ donors ourselves because I couldn't see through my tears to drive. Our laughter momentarily broke the heavy gloom, but the oppressive fear that surrounded us would remain a constant fixture in our lives for many weeks to come.

When we finally arrived at the hospital, I wondered how I would have the strength to get out of the car and walk through the entrance. I was absolutely terrified, and I marveled at how calm Doug seemed to be. I mindlessly handed my keys to the valet man, and Doug and I immediately rushed toward the hospital entrance with our hastily packed bags in tow.

I couldn't help wondering when and if Doug would feel the sunlight upon his face again. I took a deep breath and inhaled the sweetness of the warm air to calm myself. I held the air in my lungs, and I prayed that Doug would soon be able to do the same. When we walked through the revolving doors, it was as if we were passing through a portal. I wanted more than anything to believe that the portal held the promise of a new and exciting chapter in our lives. But as the sweet air of the early spring day was replaced by the stale and heavy air of the hospital, I feared that the portal might only be holding the events and words that would compose our final chapter.

We mindlessly made our way to the admissions department to officially begin the transplant journey. We were immediately seated in a small cubicle, and I nervously clutched my bag as if it held all of my worldly possessions. The secretary typed furiously on the computer while she explained parking, hotel vouchers, power of attorney, and other assorted paperwork. I was unable to process the majority of what she said, but I was astute enough to chuckle whenever she made an attempt at a joke. I wanted to find some levity in the situation in which we now found ourselves, and her spunky attempts at making us feel comfortable did provide some relief.

Unfortunately, I found myself simultaneously irritated and comforted by her humor, and my emotions vacillated madly between annoyance and amusement as I listened to her speak and watched the collection of paperwork grow. I was never so relieved when she finally allowed us to go to the transplant unit. If we were going to commit ourselves to this transplant, I wanted to do it immediately. I wanted this day to end.

When we arrived at the transplant unit, we were calmly shown to a regular hospital room. There was a short respite before Doug's coordinator entered the room to tell us that the new lungs were still looking good. This was great news, but I just wanted to go home. I hated the starkness of the hospital room, and I longed for the familiarity, warmth, and comfort of our own home. I wanted Doug to be healthy, and I wanted to go home. But I knew that I could not have my wish without the transplant.

A flurry of nurses and residents then entered the room, and I moved myself to the corner in an attempt to stay out of their way. I felt helpless and removed as I watched them work on my husband. Everything they did and said was foreign to me. Suddenly, just as quickly as they had come, they disappeared. We were alone again, and we were again overwhelmed by our emotions. We sat on the bed and held each other. My heart ached as I wondered if I would ever feel his body against mine again. There was a familiarity and comfort in his arms, and I didn't want to let go.

An anesthesiologist soon came in to explain the surgery to us. It was amazing to listen to him explain the process of the procedure. I again felt completely removed from my surroundings; I was a daydreaming student in a science lecture. I followed his words, but I had difficulty connecting the words and the procedures to my husband. This cannot be happening, my mind silently repeated. I nodded as the doctor spoke, but I just could not imagine that Doug would soon be unconscious on an operating table.

The parade of doctors, nurses, and "I don't know who's" continued over the course of the next few hours. Finally, the transplant surgeon entered the room and told us that the surgery was officially a "go." The fear that had been my companion since the early afternoon consumed me, and I immediately wanted to be sick. I can't do this. This cannot be happening. I can't let him go. But these words would never be given a voice; they would forever remain as unspoken thoughts. I looked at my husband and nodded; we were going to do this. It was happening, and we were going to let it happen.

"Are you sure that the lungs look good?" Doug asked the surgeon.

We were scared, and we were seeking assurance from the man who was about to hold Doug's life in his hands. His response bewildered us: "I've been in this business for a long time, and if you don't trust me, then maybe we shouldn't do this. I'm not going to stand here and try to sell you a pair of lungs. You are a very sick guy, and I don't know how much time you have left. If you don't want these lungs, just let me know, and we'll give them to someone else, and I'll go home and get some sleep."

We were looking for assurance, but insensitivity or some strange version of surgical tough love was the only offering. I knew that time was a precious commodity in transplantation, but I was living with the possibility that my husband might not survive the surgery. The thought that this exchange might be one of Doug's last experiences on this earth enraged me, so I fought back the emotions that were on the verge of being unhinged and entered the conversation.

"We are scared to death, and we are just looking for some reassurance. My husband wasn't questioning your ability. He just wants to hear that the lungs look really good."

The doctor glanced in my direction, but he did not respond. He looked back at Doug and repeated the question, "Do you want these lungs?"

The unanswered question hung in the air for a brief moment, and then Doug looked at me and said, "Yes, yes I want them."

We were then left alone for a few minutes until the head anesthesiologist came up to talk to Doug. She re-explained the procedure, and as she concluded her speech, I looked at Doug, and he began to weep. The anesthesiologist excused herself and told us that she would give us a few minutes.

I fell into Doug's arms, and I was certain that my heart was going to break. Every fiber of my being hurt, and I didn't know how I was going to let go of him. I searched my mind for something to say to him, but I ultimately decided that I would not make any profound professions. He knew how I felt about him, and I knew how he felt about me, and that was enough. We both feared that anything more than "I love you" would seem like a final goodbye. "I love you" seemed less daunting and lacked the finality of some overblown soliloquy. I held on to him as long as I possibly could in an attempt to memorize the feeling of his presence. I drank in his smell and prayed that I would one day be able to hold him again. "We're ready for you," the anesthesiologist said. I hated those words, but I knew that it was time.

The soul would have no rainbow had the eyes no tears.
—John Vance Cheney

Waiting with Banana Bread

The walk to the operating room was like having a tooth pulled. It was quick, but there was a throbbing pain that remained when it ended. Fortunately for Doug, he had been given a sedative, and he was more than content to take a ride on a gurney. As we traveled through the maze of hospital corridors, he chatted with the anesthesiologists and even sang a little of Joan Osborne's song "One of Us." Doug was performing a one man concert, and I couldn't help chuckling at how he had become virtually oblivious to his situation. The head anesthesiologist told me that the sedatives were working very well and that Doug would not remember any part of the journey to the operating room. I wanted to share in Doug's oblivion, and I asked her if she could give me a dose of the same medicine. She thought that I was joking, but I had never been more serious in my life.

When we reached the entrance of the operating room, I knew that it was time to say our final good-bye. My heart physically ached. I bent over to kiss him, and I said with a smile, "I'll see you later." I intentionally emphasized the word "later" in an attempt to convey a temporary parting and not an end.

Doug smiled at me and said, "Yep, see you on the other side."

I smiled tentatively at the anesthesiologist, and he sensed my fear. "Don't worry, he's in great hands," he said.

I nodded. Yes, he was indeed in very good hands. He was now in God's hands.

I suddenly found myself standing alone outside of the entrance to the operating room. The chaos of the day ended as abruptly as it had started, and I was now the lone being in the middle of a hospital hallway. I was scared and confused, and I clung to the only things that were still familiar to me: a duffle bag, a lung transplant binder, a portable oxygen tank, and Doug's shoes, coat, pants, shirt, and glasses. I noticed that the walls and the tile flooring were stark white, and the color was so cold and sterile that it intensified my loneliness. I didn't know where to go or what to do. I had been given directions to the cardiothoracic surgical waiting room, and since I had nowhere else to go, I began to make my way to yet another unfamiliar place. But as I began to walk, and the tears started to flow, I knew that I did not have the strength to wait alone.

My family and Doug's family lived out of state, and I had assumed that I would be fine until they were able to arrive. I tried to walk to the cardiothoracic waiting room, but my emotions would not allow me to complete the journey. I stopped near a garbage can, placed all of my belongings on the floor, and pulled out my cell phone. I called my brother in San Francisco and tearfully told him that the surgery was about to start, and I needed someone to come immediately. As any protective big brother would do, he quickly set about the task of arranging travel, and he and I began the process of notifying friends and relatives. But after a few calls, I gave up that task because I couldn't speak more than a few words without falling apart.

I needed a diversion, so I decided that I would try to eat something. I took all of our personal belongings back to the car and went to the cafeteria. I wandered around the cafeteria aimlessly and did my best to find some gastric delight that appeared remotely appetizing. I immediately discovered that this would not be an easy task. Everything was fried, covered in gravy, or just simply indistinguishable as a food product. I wondered if the cardiac unit and the cafeteria had arranged some sort of business deal that would ensure a constant and steady stream of patients.

I decided to be safe and delay my stay in the cardiac unit by purchasing a slice of banana bread and a carton of milk—skim milk, thank you very much. I slowly made my way back to the surgical waiting room and when I arrived, I sat down in a rocking chair and began the process of trying to choke down my cafeteria treasures.

My treasures were simple and basic, but eating them would be no simple task. Each time I took a bite of the banana bread, my stomach churned, and my mouth begged me to remove the unwelcome and offending offering. I grimaced as I drank the milk that tasted like water that had been sitting in a cardboard box for two weeks. But I knew that my mind and body needed nutrition, so I continued to force feed myself until the rumbling of a gag signaled the end of my culinary adventure.

Meanwhile, my cell phone kept ringing, and I was thrilled by the thought of being connected to someone familiar each time it rang. When my mom called, all of my emotion was finally unhinged. Through my sobbing, I was finally able to articulate exactly what I was feeling, "I don't think I'm strong enough to do this." I was thirty-five years old, and I wanted my mommy.

As I waited for our family to arrive, the day quickly turned to night. I watched the sun go down like a curtain closing at the end of a Broadway performance, and I prayed that this day's curtain would not signal an end, but a new beginning. I couldn't help wondering what life altering changes the sun's rising curtain would reveal the following morning.

Our future had never been certain, and this fact was magnified by my solitude and the darkness that had now overtaken the day. The darkness of night always intensifies and stirs the fears that lie dormant in our minds, and fear comes so easily and naturally when our thoughts are our only companions.

So the darkness that blanketed my world and the solitude of the waiting room naturally and quickly became my worst enemies. My mind was free to roam, and it unfortunately chose to roam toward fear. Did I even dare to think of the wonderful possibilities that this transplant could bring? I was too afraid to look forward. Making plans and thinking of the boundless possibilities seemed presumptuous, and I feared that my hopes would be dashed if I basked in their presence for too long.

I tried to divert my attention away from my thoughts and fears. The waiting room was in front of a large window that overlooked one of the hospital's helicopter landing pads, and I watched with great anticipation for the helicopter that might be carrying my husband's new lungs. One helicopter did arrive, but I was disappointed when I saw an empty gurney being wheeled toward it.

I tried to watch TV, but I was unable to focus. I spent several hours staring aimlessly outside while attempting to soothe myself with the motion of the rocking chair. Doug had given me his wedding ring before he was taken to surgery, and I stared at it and held it tightly as I begged God for his life. The hours were passing slowly, and I was relieved when a friend called to tell me that she and another friend were going to drive over to sit with me until my family arrived.

After sitting alone for four hours, my two friends finally arrived. It was like seeing water in the desert. I was no longer alone, and I immediately felt stronger and more confident. An hour after their arrival, I was told that the doctors had removed one lung, transplanted one of the new lungs, and were beginning the process of removing the second lung. I was relieved to hear the news, and I began to cling to this tiny piece of hope. I was still lost in a sea of emotion, but this news felt like a life preserver that just might have the ability to sustain me.

My friends and I sat together for three more hours before I saw the transplant surgeon come through the doors toward the waiting room. I saw him immediately, and I searched his eyes for answers. He held my gaze as he walked toward me, but his facial expression did not change. He looked stoic, and my heart began to race, as I feared the worst. After eight hours of waiting, I heard the words that I had craved, "The surgery went well." I was relieved and elated to hear that I would be able to see Doug in less than an hour. He had survived the surgery, and I slowly began to allow myself to consider the possibility of a successful transplant.

The message of dawn is hope.
—*Winston Churchill*

The Circle of Life

Doug's sister arrived shortly after the surgery had ended, and she was able to accompany me to see Doug for the first time in the ICU about an hour after they had brought him back from the operating room. I was scared as I walked into the room, but I was desperate to see his face again. When I stepped into the room, I was shocked at the number of machines, tubes, and IV lines that were connected to him. The scene was visually and audibly overwhelming, and I struggled to maintain my composure.

I immediately noticed a loud gurgling noise that emanated from two briefcase-sized boxes at the foot of his bed. These boxes were collection chambers for fluid and blood that were connected to his four chest tubes. Meanwhile, the ventilator contributed a rhythmic and bizarrely soothing hiss to the entire scene. His nurse worked diligently as she raced around his bed adjusting lines and hanging IV bags while never losing her focus on the two monitors that tracked his vital signs. The room was overwhelming, but my Doug was alive, and despite all of the tubes and lines, he looked strangely healthy and peaceful.

I stared at him and held his hand. In an attempt to soothe myself, I stroked his forehead repetitively, and I ran my fingers through the hair that I had cropped too short just a few days before. He looked helpless, and although his body was present, he seemed so far away. I wanted desperately to see his eyes and hear his voice, but I knew that I had to be satisfied with this first step. I looked up to talk to his sister, but she had already left the room. Visions of Doug as a child had flashed through her mind as she looked at him, and she quickly became overwhelmed. Doug and I were alone, and I would stay by his side as long as the nurses would allow.

As I familiarized myself with Doug's new home, I quickly became fixated with the monitor above his bed that was filled with colorful lines and numbers. I knew that these numbers and lines represented life, and I was elated to watch their beautifully choreographed dance on the screen. But I also knew that the next forty-eight hours were critical as the doctors and nurses would continually scan every vital sign for signs of complications and organ rejection, and the fear that I had felt all day continued its relentless hold on me.

I went back out to the waiting room and tried to sleep on the waiting room couch. But sleep would be elusive. I spent the next four hours shivering under a light blanket and staring at images of the war with Iraq on the TV screen. My eyes darted between the TV and the doors that led to the entrance of Doug's hospital wing. The doors were automatic, and they made a loud and repetitive noise every time they opened.

I quickly learned to loathe those doors and their accompanying sound, as they began to symbolize the fear and uncertainty of the experience. I never knew what was going on behind them, or who was going to pass through them. I cautiously watched every doctor who walked through those doors and let out a sigh of relief when he or she would pass by the waiting room. I viewed every person dressed in a white coat as a potential bearer of bad news. But there would be no bad news that early morning, and the next few hours would reunite me with more family and friends. I was no longer alone, Doug was alive, and our transplant journey was underway.

Doug would spend the next twenty-five days in the hospital, and each day would bring a new joy. Unfortunately, each new joy was often accompanied by a new and unexpected battle. His first battle began the day after his transplant when he developed a re-implantation response or reperfusion edema: a complication which occurs due to a lack of blood flow and oxygen to the new lungs. The result is that the swollen lungs are unable to provide sufficient oxygenation to the body, and the patient must receive treatment that includes inhaled nitric oxide and extracorporeal membrane oxygenation (ECMO). In simple terms, ECMO mechanically oxygenates the blood, which thereby eliminates the burden on the lungs and allows them to heal. It was frightening to hear that Doug's lungs were not functioning properly, but I was sleep deprived and emotionally drained, and the doctor's words seemed to fall harmlessly upon my numb body.

The first time I saw Doug after he was placed on the ECMO machine, I was astonished. The machine was very large, and since his room was already brimming with machinery, there was virtually no room to maneuver around his bed. I was immediately entranced by the two long tubes that crept surreptitiously from under the sheets to snake their way to the ECMO machine. The tubes were clear and surprisingly large, and it was clearly evident which tube carried the unoxygenated blood away from his body and which tube carried the oxygenated blood back into his body. The oxygenated blood was a vivid shade of red, while the unoxygenated blood was a strikingly dark and dull shade of the same color. I thought about how appropriate it was that the blood which carried the life sustaining oxygen was so vibrantly rich and red. When you take time to truly see the color palette of life, the colors are vibrant and striking, and the tube that carried the life sustaining blood back to my husband was brimming with that same vibrancy.

Doug remained on the ECMO machine for two days. It was pure joy to see the machine removed from his room and to know that he had crossed a very big hurdle. It had been four days since his surgery, and since he was no longer dependent upon the ECMO machine, the doctors began the process of waking him.

I will never forget the morning when I called the hospital at 5:00 a.m. to find out how Doug had fared during the night. The nurse told me that Doug was finally awake. My heart skipped a beat, and I quickly went about the business of getting ready to go see him. I flew down to my brother and father's hotel room to tell them the news, and we then quickly hurried to make our way to the hospital. I was elated and excited, but the three-minute drive to the hospital in the hotel shuttle seemed to take an eternity.

It was a cold and snowy Wisconsin morning, and winter was making its final stand. The brisk air took my breath away, and I raised the collar of my coat and burrowed myself into the car's seat in an attempt to beat away the early morning cold that tugged at me. The warmth of the car slowly began to surround me, and I was flooded with the memories of the bright and sunny spring day that had led us to this point only four days earlier. But that day was now reduced to a distant memory, and the snowflakes that fell gently upon the van's windshield seemed to distance the memory even more.

When we arrived at the hospital, I scurried up to the fifth floor. Part of the ICU's routine mandated that I call from the waiting room before entering Doug's room. I picked up the phone and spoke the words that had become programmed in my brain, "This is Doug Broehl's wife. Is it okay for me to visit him now?" There was always a pause that was followed by indistinguishable banter and noise. "Yes, come right in; he's asking for you." My mind was shocked by this unexpected news, and my heart soared. Doug was finally awake, and he was asking for me.

I rushed to his room with my mind brimming with anticipation. And when I finally saw his face, I felt an overwhelming sense of peace, joy, and inexplicable gratitude. He looked peaceful, and his skin had a gloriously pink glow that radiated a healthy and youthful exuberance. But the peacefulness that surrounded him would suddenly and unexpectedly disappear as he contorted his face in pain as he tried to move or swallow. My heart broke for him as I could sense his discomfort.

The breathing tube that connected to the ventilator was especially unpleasant, and I felt helpless to make things better for him. But he never moved his head away from my direction, and I knew that my presence helped to ease his pain. He tried desperately to focus his eyes upon me, but he was unable to see my face clearly. He seemed to be looking at me, but there was a distance in his eyes, and his gaze seemed to pass right through me. I moved closer to his face, but it was to no avail. He would initially have to settle for the comfort and familiarity of my voice.

I stared at him, and I was mesmerized by the sight of his eyes as I struggled to read the emotion and thoughts hidden behind them. I saw a tear slowly roll down his face, and I was certain that he was sharing my joy. He was alive, I could talk to him, and he could squeeze my hand. Nothing else mattered as I basked in the living presence of my husband.

Doug continued to progress rapidly, and I was amazed by his strength. His once lifeless body was quickly replaced by a body that craved movement and freedom. He moved his arms and legs about restlessly and tried desperately to communicate. He would attempt to mouth words, but the breathing tube made it virtually impossible to read his lips. He attempted to write words on a clipboard, but the writing was completely illegible. The poorly written words flowed together, and I was left to decipher several sheets of paper that resembled a psychiatrist's collection of Rorschach cards. Absolutely nothing would dissuade him from communicating. He wanted to know about his health, his family, and his friends, but just hearing about these things would not be enough. He also wanted to talk.

Doug is a man of many thoughts and ideas, and a ventilator was not going to change that fact. He would try to mouth words, and he would use his hands to perform a crude rendition of sign language. I could see the desperation and frustration in his eyes, but I could rarely understand him, and I often lacked the ability and insight to guess what he wanted. My emotional stress level and the lack of sleep made communicating with him all the more difficult. This routine continued for five exhausting days, and as my frustration level grew along with his, I asked God to give me the patience that I would surely need to endure this challenge.

The breathing tube also made it impossible for him to swallow, and as a result, his mouth was very dry, and he craved any source of moisture. I was able to give him water via a mouth swab, and he delighted in putting the swab between his cheek and gums and sucking every drop of water from it. His eyes would close, and a look of peacefulness and pure contentment would settle upon his face. But the satisfaction he felt was fleeting.

The water that provided so much relief would then have to be suctioned from his mouth, and the dryness that he so desperately wanted to eliminate would quickly return. It was a vicious and unrelenting circle, and my new role as a water girl was exhausting. But peace, joy, and relief would be ours shortly. Nine days after his transplant, the doctors decided to remove the breathing tube and shut down the ventilator.

The day the breathing tube was removed was one of the best days of my life. I will never have the experience of giving birth, but I was able to witness the birth of a new life on April 9, 2003. When the respiratory therapist pulled Doug's breathing tube, I heard a short and quick gasp. I looked down at Doug's chest and saw it moving up and down, and I realized that he was breathing completely on his own. There was no ventilator, and there was no ECMO machine. His lungs were functioning perfectly on their own.

It was miraculous to watch him breathe, and I was overcome with emotion. I leaned over his bed to be closer to his face, and I saw the tears of joy silently cascade down his face and fall harmlessly upon his pillow. I asked him if he was in pain or if his tears were tears of happiness. He tried to talk, but his voice was weak and hoarse. Nevertheless, I could easily distinguish the first word that he spoke to me, "Happy."

I laid my head on his shoulder, and we cried tears of pure joy and utter relief. And somewhere within those tears of joy, I cried tears of sadness for Doug's donor and his family. My heart ached for this unknown family's loss, and I was simultaneously overwhelmed by the incredible joy that they had unselfishly given to us that day. The circle of life was complete, and it was reflected in every tear that fell.

I command you—be strong and courageous! Do not be afraid or discouraged. For the Lord your God is with you wherever you go.

—Joshua 1:9 (NLT)

Moving Forward

After the breathing tube was removed, Doug was immediately taken out of his bed and put into an old lime green hospital chair. It was odd to see him sitting upright, and his confused facial expression echoed my sentiments. The respiratory therapists immediately began his breathing treatments, and Doug was given the task of trying to hold onto an oversized nebulizer that had a tendency to gyrate uncontrollably. His hands were weak, and he struggled to hold it while keeping his body upright in the chair. I felt sorry for him, and I wanted to help him. But I knew that this was the beginning of the slow and arduous process of returning to life after a transplant. This battle was his, and I would have to leave him to fight it.

Each day brought new joys and challenges for Doug. His first and greatest joy was found in a can of Coke. After being on the ventilator for nine days, Doug was anxious to drink something. Unfortunately, the doctors had to restrict him to ice chips and water from a mouth swab for the first several hours after his breathing tube was removed. But it was not long before a nurse brought him a can of Coke and instructed him to take small sips and swallow slowly. Doug gingerly cradled the can of soda and began the process of trying to place his lips around the straw that danced away from his mouth every time he approached it. When his lips finally locked on the straw, and the sugary brown liquid rose to his mouth, a look of absolute delight and relief crossed Doug's face. His face lit up, and he exclaimed, "Oh my God, this is the best thing that I have ever tasted in my life." I giggled at his reaction, and we smiled at one another as we savored the pure simplicity and joy of the moment. Doug could breathe with ease for the first time in years, but he was much more enthralled and delighted by his can of Coke.

Doug's first meal after his surgery was equally entertaining. It was a liquid meal, but in his eyes, it was a four-course extravaganza from a gourmet restaurant. His hospital tray was brimming with a bowl of pureed vegetable beef soup, strawberry sherbet, butterscotch pudding, a can of Coke, and apple juice. His hands were unsteady and weak, so I assumed the task of feeding him. I would scoop up the food, and he would anxiously move forward in his chair with his mouth wide open. He reminded me of a baby bird that eagerly anticipates its mother and her gift of food. Thankfully, we are not birds, so I did not have to chew the food and spit it into his mouth.

When the food hit his tongue for the first time, his body crumpled back into his chair, and he nodded his head and groaned at the sheer delight of eating, tasting, and swallowing again. In all honesty, he looked like he was having a small seizure. Each time he would eat something, his head would start bobbing, and he would loudly exclaim, "Oh my God. Oh my God. This is so good. Oh my God, Dana. This tastes incredible." I couldn't wait to scoop up some more food, as his litany of joy became like a broken record. He couldn't get enough food, and I couldn't shovel it in fast enough. When the tray was finally littered with the remnants of his feast, he looked at me with a slightly scrunched face and said, "I think I ate too much." I was afraid that he might vomit, but he just sat back in his chair and grinned, full of the satisfaction of a good meal.

Doug's stay in the ICU was also full of difficult and dark moments. Shortly after the breathing tube was removed, he began to experience ICU psychosis. This is a condition which is characterized by strange dreams and hallucinations and is most commonly caused by a combination of sensory deprivation, sleep disturbances, and medication.

Doug's psychosis manifested itself in visions of Dante's Inferno. He spoke repetitively of hell, and he perceived every doctor as an enemy. He saw flames emanating from the doctors' eyes and mouths, and their presence was always sure to agitate him. He even began to perceive his morphine as evil, and he referred to it as "the enemy." He would often refuse to take it, but the nurses and I were slowly able to convince him that morphine was not the devil's drug. I wanted to strangle Dante and his Godforsaken book.

Doug was also very childlike. He would sit in his room and stare at his surroundings in much the same way that a newborn examines his or her new world. His focus would flutter aimlessly and unpredictably. He would drift miles away while staring at various objects in the room, and then just as quickly as he had drifted away, he would suddenly propel himself back into the land of the living by engaging in a seemingly endless stream of semi-coherent conversation. There was just too much for him to take in and understand all at once, and his senses were tainted by the immune-suppressing drug cocktail that he consumed like a sailor on a drunken binge. I had had nine days to begin to adjust to this new world, and my mind was not clouded by pharmaceuticals.

Everything was new to Doug, and he struggled to comprehend his new surroundings and reality. He had a new pair of lungs and a new ability to breath, but this new ability was coupled with an inability to move and control his muscles at will. His muscles had been weakened by the surgery and the extended period of inactivity, and he needed to retrain and recondition them. His body had been his companion for thirty-eight years, and everything that was once comfortable and known was now uncomfortable and foreign.

Doug's first physical challenge was to walk. Twelve days after his transplant, a therapist entered his room and announced that it was time to start walking. I gazed around the room and looked at the unending number of cords and tubes that were still attached to Doug, and I quietly wondered how walking could even be considered as a possibility. But like a master magician, the therapist began the process of moving, unhooking, and transferring cords, and it was not long before a dazed Doug was on his feet.

Doug held on to a wheelchair while the therapist gently cradled his waist for support. The scene was slightly chaotic, so I was given the simple task of trailing behind with the IV pole. We had become a three-person circus parade that was about to make its way onto the streets of the hospital.

Doug's first steps were painfully slow and deliberate, but he was walking. My duty as IV girl was slow and tedious, so I began to sing the words of one of my favorite childhood songs in my head. "Put one foot in front of the other, and soon you'll be walking across the floor. Put one foot in front of the other, and soon you'll be walking out the door." The song helped me to pass the time, and it lessened the sting of watching my thirty-eight-year-old husband struggle to walk again.

Doug was able to walk out of his room and around the short hallway of the ICU. His pace was excruciatingly slow, but after twelve days in a hospital bed, he felt like he was flying at the speed of light. When we returned to the room, Doug was beaming with pride. "I did it, Dana. I walked." He gingerly sat down in the same chair that had cradled his battered body immediately after his breathing tube was pulled, and for the next several minutes he smiled and nodded at his tremendous accomplishment. He looked up at me, his blue eyes hazy with tears, and exclaimed, "I really did it. I really walked."

Among the many physical challenges, Doug also had to adjust to his new lungs. The sounds were different, and the feeling was different. His old lungs had always crackled and groaned under the weight of the constant infections, but these new lungs were eerily clear and silent. Their silence was frightening for Doug, but the new sounds that would occasionally emanate from these two strangers was even more disconcerting.

One day, Doug heard a gurgling noise, and he automatically assumed that the gurgling would be a prelude to a lung bleed. He franticly asked me, "Is there blood? Am I coughing up blood?" I calmly reminded him that he now had new lungs; lungs that would not bleed unexpectedly like his old ones. "These are good lungs, Doug. Trust them," I said. But learning to read and trust his body would be a difficult and unnerving process.

As a result of all of the medication and physical changes, Doug was very unsure of himself and needed constant reassurance. He was afraid of being left alone, and he was afraid of sleeping. I spent thirteen to fourteen hours a day by his bedside trying to comfort and console him, but I often felt like a failure.

I cursed myself for not buying those damn Tony Robbins' tapes and books that I constantly saw on TV as I channel surfed. I had always belittled his ridiculously overpriced self-help series, but I couldn't help thinking that Tony Robbins would be better suited for the position in which I now found myself. Nevertheless, I did my best to encourage Doug and talk him through his most difficult moments. I even wrote a list of positive affirmations that he could read during the middle of the night while I was at the hotel. Who needed Tony Robbins anyway? I had a pen and a piece of paper, and I could write sentences that dripped with self-affirming encouragement.

Despite my best efforts, Doug continued to struggle, and it was difficult to watch him in this state because I ultimately knew that there was so little that I could do to soothe him. He was irrational and behaved in a manner that was completely out of character. My husband had become a complete stranger to me, and I anxiously wondered when and if my real husband would return. But with each day that passed, he grew less agitated, had fewer hallucinations, and finally began to see reality. Doug was a caterpillar that was about to emerge from his cocoon to become the butterfly that would soon spread his wings and fly.

Doug was released from the ICU two weeks after his transplant. I was elated that he was healthy and stable enough to be moved to a regular room, but the truth be told, I was more elated by the fact that we would finally be able to leave the ICU room. Doug's room in the ICU had become a prison cell, and we were its prisoners.

The room was actually quite large by hospital standards, but the walls were painted in the obligatory shade of institutional white, and the cold and colorless tile flooring enhanced and completed the depressing scenario. There was a tiny window tucked in the corner of the room that offered virtually no daylight or sunlight, and Doug's bed was positioned in such a manner that he couldn't even see the paltry view that it offered. Surprisingly, of all of the things that agitated Doug, the room was not one of them.

I had grown to hate the stark room and its many unpleasant memories, and I prayed for new surroundings. What I really wanted was a birthing suite. I wondered why pregnant women were the only people who were privy to the land of hospital suites. I tried to understand the logic: if you can squeeze a watermelon through a tiny hole, then you are entitled to a birthing suite. But if you are cut in half and have an organ removed and replaced, then you are entitled to a cold and crappy institutional walk-in closet. When I become queen of the world, my first priority will be to enact a law that grants hospital suites to all transplant patients. For that matter, anyone who must endure a hospital stay should be given a suite. It is the only decent thing to do.

Doug was moved to a room that had a gloriously large window that overlooked a city street. I was thrilled to have a window, and I was thrilled to see signs of life outside of the hospital. The cars and the people who bustled outside of this window taunted us with the freedom that eluded our grasp, but the view also served as an encouraging reminder that the land of the living continued to move forward. We were inching closer to freedom, and we knew that it was only a matter of time until we would be able to move forward and become a part of the world that we could now only watch from the hospital window.

What I failed to notice in my excitement was the fact that the window faced the west and overlooked the hospital's main helicopter landing pad. I have two words to describe our new environment: hot and noisy.

Despite the tremendous amount of noise that it created and the characteristic smell of diesel that it left behind as its calling card, the helicopter was an exciting diversion. But the afternoon sun was completely devoid of any redeeming qualities. The heat in the room would quickly escalate, and Doug and I found ourselves playing the role of the cake in a room that felt like a child's Easy-Bake Oven. We threw blankets over the windows, complained to each other about how hot we were, and laughed at the non-oscillating six-inch fan that we were given to combat the heat. Thankfully, our suffering was not destined to last, as we were blessed with a delightful string of cloudy days that put an end to our days in the Easy-Bake Oven.

The remaining days in the hospital were filled with chest x-rays, blood tests, bronchoscopies, physical therapy, cardiopulmonary rehabilitation, and lessons on new medication. Doug was now required to take sixteen different prescription medications, and each one had to be taken at a very specific time. He had to learn their names, dosages, purposes, and most importantly, their dosing schedule.

Shortly after Doug was moved out of the ICU, his sixteen drugs were delivered to the room in a pink vomit basin. It was the perfect apparatus: it held all of the medication and could easily catch a bundle of vomit at a moment's notice. Our little pink vomit bucket became our constant companion, and the habit of shoveling through it to unearth the medicine of the hour became a programmed routine.

Each day someone would enter the room and begin the process of teaching something new. The closet that was called a hospital room quickly became cluttered with the teaching materials that each person would bring, and our minds were becoming cluttered with their facts, figures, and expectations. Doug's brain was slowed by painkillers and anti-anxiety medication, and my mind was dulled from the accumulating lack of sleep, but we still managed to process everything that was tossed our way. Doug had to know his medication schedule in order to be released from the hospital, and so we quickly became diligent students and devoured and memorized any information that was given to us. We were not going to let anything prevent our escape from the hospital that was becoming our own personal Alcatraz.

Doug continued to grow stronger with the passing of each day, and the boredom that filled our lives made each day seem like an eternity. Each day became indistinguishable from the previous day, and time slowly blended into a haze. There was so little excitement in our lives that the highlight of my existence became Taco Tuesdays in the hospital cafeteria. We felt like lab rats that were being observed for some perverse psychological test. We walked, talked, played cards, and stared aimlessly at the four walls that seemed to be progressively closing in on us.

We logically knew that Doug was one of the lucky transplant patients. He had survived his surgery, and his hospital stay had been relatively easy and brief. But the emotional magnitude of the experience robbed us of our ability to put things in perspective, and immersing ourselves in our own little world of self-pity and frustration became a comfortable and safe place. Our focus became freedom. We wanted out of the hospital, and empathy and understanding for other patients were non-existent.

We were finally given a release date, but that date was eventually delayed by a surprise fungal infection. We began to fear that freedom would never be ours and that the evil fungal infection would dash our new dreams, but on April 24, 2003, twenty-five days after his transplant, Doug was finally discharged from the hospital. We would have to live in a nearby hotel for the next week, but the freedom and privacy that we had craved since his admission would now be ours.

Enjoy the little things, for one day you may look back and realize they were the big things.

—Robert Brault

Inching toward a Life

Living in a hotel was wonderful—for the first few days. There were no doctors, residents, medical students, x-ray technicians, phlebotomists, nurses, physical therapists, or janitors to parade through the room, and we were no longer bombarded by the unrelenting sounds and smells of a hospital.

In our new hotel home, the distinctive smell of institutional food no longer wafted into the room three times a day, occluded IV lines no longer screamed for attention, and the dreaded floor cleaning machine that resembled an ice rink Zamboni no longer rumbled down the hallway leaving the pungent smell of dusty lemons in its wake.

Instead, we found ourselves in an alarmingly quiet hotel room that oozed polyester fabrics, simulated wood grain furniture, garishly colored bedspreads, and carpeting that resembled colorful vomit. It was a synthetic paradise, and we were thrilled to be basking in its visually stimulating glory.

During our first night of freedom, we engaged in the simple pleasure of going to Target and a local restaurant for carryout pasta. It was an amazing venture, and it was incredible how such a simple outing could be so ridiculously pleasurable. Freedom and health had given us a new perspective and appreciation for life, and even the most mundane tasks seemed richer and more pleasant that day. Waiting at stoplights and standing in checkout lines were no longer chores; they were joyful acts that lose their meaning among the healthy.

When we returned to the hotel, we were thrilled to eat dinner on a hotel desk that we had turned into a makeshift dining room table. After eating hospital food for nearly a month, the simple fast-food pasta dishes tasted as if they had been prepared by a gourmet Italian chef. The food melted in our mouths, and the divine taste momentarily transported us to a lovely and quaint little Venetian bistro at the river's edge. But we were in a poorly decorated room that swirled with the noise of the freeway that ran along the edge of the hotel, and on that glorious evening, our small room in Madison, Wisconsin was just as appealing as the Venetian bistro that existed in our minds.

We talked a little, but the majority of the dinner was filled with the sounds of moaning as we feasted on heavenly food that burst with real flavor. "Oh my God, this is so good. This is just absolutely incredible. My mouth hasn't experienced this much joy in a month." Between the moaning and our running commentary during the meal, I'm quite certain that anyone who may have overheard us must have thought that our room was a passion pit. But there was only passion and tremendous love for our bountiful plates of pasta.

We spent nine days in the hotel, and although Doug was free from the hospital, we were certainly not leading independent lives. We were the children of an institution that refused to cut the apron strings. There was still lab work, chest x-rays, bronchoscopies, and cardiopulmonary rehabilitation to be done.

I hated driving back to the hospital after he was discharged because I feared that each time we stepped foot in the place, the doctors would discover some new problem and reclaim him as theirs. He was mine again, and I wanted to keep it that way. I began to develop a slight disdain for the place that had saved my husband's life; I wanted to wrestle free from the firm grip that it insisted on maintaining.

Whenever the oversized brown hospital complex came into my line of sight, a slight sneer would automatically cross my face, and my left nostril would slowly flare while the left side of my upper lip would levitate. I had become angry Elvis, and I only needed a peanut butter and banana sandwich and a sequined jumpsuit to complete my metamorphosis.

After our hospital commitments were completed in the morning, the remnant of the day was ours. Since we had always enjoyed the enticing allure of any and every bookstore, we usually chose to spend the afternoon among the shelves and stacks of endless literary jewels. There was a familiarity and comfort in bookstores, and we loved to pass the time enveloped in the smell of newly published books and freshly brewed coffee. Each time we would go, we would carefully select our precious cargo and then find a cozy corner to lose ourselves among the words and the pages.

Doug would always choose one academic title, and I would flit around the store as I struggled to choose my distraction. I would inevitably feel shallow and guilty when I would return to the corner with my stack of celebrity and decorating magazines. Doug was devouring information on how the philosophy of the Classical age influenced Beethoven, and I was reading about the challenges of decorating a small space. But I still craved simplicity, and my intellectually light fare was more than satisfying. I was a walking vessel of useless information. I was the American dream.

We also went to every shopping mall in the city, and we could have easily become culinary critics based on the number of restaurants we frequented. Freedom was sweet, the food was even sweeter, Doug grew physically stronger by the day, and the phrase "There just aren't enough hours in the day" quickly became meaningless and incomprehensible to us. There were plenty of hours in the day, and time often seemed to grind to a screeching halt. So it was no surprise that the droning boredom that had become such a predominant presence in the hospital slowly began to creep back into our lives.

We were ready to move on to the next phase of our lives, but the doctors were not ready to release Doug and his fungal infection from the safety and confines of the city. We knew that staying in Madison was in Doug's best interest, but logic and rational understanding offered little consolation, and they certainly didn't soothe the beastly boredom.

When the doctors finally made the decision to allow us to go home, I had imagined a feeling of pure elation. I imagined myself flying out of the hotel with reckless abandon, and I feared for any man, woman, or child who might make the fatal error of getting in my way as I bolted through the doors of freedom. But I was surprised to discover that the overwhelming excitement that I had eagerly anticipated did not materialize. I was mildly thrilled by the prospect of going home, but my meager levels of anticipation and excitement were coupled with a fairly substantial fear.

Doug and I knew that we had become two very different people after his transplant, but we did not know exactly how we were different. Each day we would engage ourselves in the process of sorting out how we had changed and what those changes would mean for our relationship. We discussed our feelings and emotions, but processing our experiences was often a confusing, difficult, and sometimes fruitless endeavor that made the thought of returning home and resuming our old lives seemed like a frightening and daunting task. We had a home, jobs, and a daily routine before his transplant, but those things had been reduced to distant and foreign memories to which we could no longer relate.

I knew that our new life would be better, but there was no familiarity in this new life; it was a complete stranger. Doug was now an able-bodied and healthy individual, and I knew that some of the dynamics and patterns that we had developed over the years would naturally need to be re-crafted. The predictability, certainty, and security that I expected Doug's new lungs to bring were accompanied by new challenges and a mountain of uncertainty. Would Doug's health continue to be the primary focus of our lives? How would our lives be different? Would our relationship change?

Going home meant that we would have to finally discover what those new challenges and uncertainties would truly be. Our journey to this point had been filled with uncertainty, and going home would not signal an end, but rather a new beginning to the unknown. The hospital had offered a strange sense of security, but now the security blanket had been removed, and we were suddenly exposed and thrust into our new future.

Where is home? Home is where the heart can laugh without shyness. Home is where the heart's tears can dry at their own pace.

—Vernon G. Baker

Home

Our return home was relatively uneventful. We traveled down the same highway that had initially led us to our journey, and I was immediately struck by the weather. The sky was brilliantly blue, and the sun shone brightly. The day was a mirror image of our first trip to Madison. But unlike that first trip, spring was now in full bloom, and winter had finally succumbed to new life. The grass was green, the flowers were blooming, and the trees carried their full load of spring's majesty. But this trip would be different. This time, we welcomed the final destination.

The house looked just as we had left it, and it was strange to reflect upon the last time we were together in our home when we were franticly trying to get ready to go to the hospital. But the journey had now come full circle, Doug was alive and well, and we were home again. We immediately collected our cat from my girlfriend's house, and we began the process of re-entering our world. But we soon discovered that picking up the pieces and returning to normalcy would be no easy task.

Doug and I felt dazed and confused by the emotions that inundated us after we returned home. We were exhausted and overwhelmed by the emotional roller coaster ride of the past month, and we vacillated between euphoric highs and lows. Doug was able to breathe freely for the first time in years, and his new lease on life rekindled the flame of hope for our future. Everything in our world seemed sweeter and more vibrant, and we were overwhelmed by our good fortune. But while our happiness was intoxicating, fear had an equal presence in our home.

Doug was still battling a fungal infection, and the issue of organ rejection was a constant and frightening presence. Despite the fact that he had yet to experience a rejection episode, the hospital had virtually tattooed the warning signs of rejection on his forehead. They also made us repeat the transplant mantra at least ten times a day: "Rejection can occur at anytime, rejection can occur at anytime. Call the transplant coordinator immediately if there are any significant changes in breathing, blood pressure, or temperature." We had been indoctrinated into the transplant cult, and leaving was not an option. There would be no deprogramming; we were members for life.

The hospital had prepared us so well that we were initially afraid to delight too much in our happiness. We worried about the unknown and the unexpected that seemed to be lurking around every corner, and we began to see shadows where there were none. Chronic illness had taught us to be cautious, and that caution was now trying to rob us of our joy.

The difficult readjustment period was also heightened by the fact that Doug was in a Prednisone haze. Prednisone is a miraculously evil drug that is used to combat rejection, but the side effects can include such pleasantries as insomnia, irritability, and mood swings. As a result, Doug was often needy and frightened, and he could easily go from laughter to tears within minutes.

I felt helpless to make things better for him, and I began to seriously wonder if I was in over my head. I would talk to him incessantly, but my words would only soothe him temporarily. He paced around the house like a caged animal lamenting his reality. He wanted to come out of his skin, and I was growing weary of the unpredictability and sadness of the stranger who was living in our home.

Doug's moodiness came to a climax one morning at 2:00 a.m. He was having difficulty sleeping, and he was pacing frantically around our bedroom. He was rambling, and he was completely inconsolable.

I woke up and tried to clear the cobwebs in my head so that I could deal with the chaos that was now confronting me in the dark. I tried to console him, but there was nothing that I could say or do to bring him peace.

In utter despair, he finally sat down on the bed and cried. Nothing could have prepared me for what he was about to say: "I wish I had never had this transplant." I was shocked, hurt, and angry. His words struck the core of my heart, and I was rendered speechless. I knew that the medication had silenced the real Doug; his words did not represent his true feelings. But logic would not comfort me. I was exhausted, and I was emotionally empty.

I remembered everything that we had gone through during the past month, and I reflected upon the endless hours that I sat at his bedside and prayed for his life. The journey had been difficult, and I was anxiously ready to move forward. My husband was healthy and alive, and I had everything that I wanted. But Doug was lost in a world that offered him no happiness or consolation. His medication would simply not allow him to savor the same joy and relief that I was feeling about his transplant. He finally had healthy lungs, but his emotions were now trapped in a tortured mind. I sat silently in bed and let the tears of frustration and disappointment silently fall while Doug finally calmed down and drifted off to sleep.

I wondered where the promise of our new and glorious life was. We had visions and dreams of what our life would be like after Doug's transplant. Doug and I would be healthy and happy, and the world would be our oyster. I imagined leisurely walks in the park surrounded by butterflies and birds while the music of a light and delicious symphony swirled in the background. We would finally be free to travel and live our lives in ways that we couldn't even begin to imagine. The possibilities were absolutely limitless.

The first few months after Doug's transplant did not offer us a carefree or simple life. We had heard the old medical cliché that getting a new organ is like trading one disease for another, but conceptualizing that reality is very different from living it. Doug could not drive, his medical routine was more complex than it was before the transplant, we had to make frequent trips to the hospital for tests and procedures, and now his mind was tortured by the very medication that kept him alive.

Doug felt tremendous gratitude for his gift of life, but that gratitude was often mingled with and overshadowed by an overwhelming sense of frustration and anger. The barriers that limited our lives before Doug's transplant were still in place, and we still felt like chained prisoners of a chronic illness. We were disillusioned, and there were days when the transplant felt more like a curse than a blessing. But we did our best to hold fast to the dream that we would soon experience the freedom that was temporarily eluding us.

Doug's mood swings were eventually tamed by anti-anxiety medication, but his personality was still different. The Prednisone had erased many of Doug's personality traits. The new Doug was a somber man who rarely laughed or smiled, and he often seemed lost in his own world. I wanted to help him, but his world was one in which I could not and did not want to be a participant. I was shocked by the irony of the situation in which I found myself. My dreams had come true, and I had a husband who could breathe again. But this man with the new lungs was a stranger to me. I wanted and expected everything, but I had no choice but to patiently await the reduction of his Prednisone and his return to me.

While I awaited Doug's return, I went back to work. There were only three weeks remaining in the semester, and I wanted to have some closure to the school year. I had spent seven months with my students, and I wanted to finish the year with them. I was also searching for some sort of distraction, and I knew that working with hormonally energetic teenagers could fulfill that role perfectly.

It was strange to open the door to my classroom and walk in for the first time in almost two months. Everything looked the same, and the familiar smell of chalk dust and books greeted me like an old friend. There was a comfortable familiarity that soothed me and made me feel like my life just might return to me. As I unpacked my book bag and continued to scan the room, I was immediately drawn to the organ donation poster that I had hung a few months before Doug's transplant. I smiled at the poster, and I momentarily enjoyed the selfish smugness of our transplant success. Doug had new lungs, and I was back at work. Life was indeed very sweet.

My first day back was wonderful, but it was also very difficult. My mind was mush, and I wandered around in a simulated drunken stupor. I felt like I had been passed out in the corner of my classroom for the past two months, and I had just awoken to discover that I had classes that still needed to be taught. My lessons were unpolished that day, and I felt completely out of synch. I even managed to botch the explanation of a grammatical concept to my Spanish V class.

I had never made such a huge mistake in my thirteen years of teaching, and while it annoyed me, I was able to quickly move past my error. I was a calmer person after Doug's transplant, and I was not going to waste time stewing over something that could be easily remedied the following day. Despite my pedagogical blunders, it was great to see my students, and I appreciated the warmth with which they greeted my return. There were smiles, hugs, and kind words all around, and I knew that I was valued and missed.

For the first time in weeks, the transplant did not rule my every thought, and the worry and fear that had clung to me began to melt away. I was able to sit in the faculty lounge and talk and laugh with my co-workers, and we even relived the day in which I had received Doug's phone call about the transplant. People were amazed at the miracle of Doug's lungs, and they felt privileged to have been in the room when that unforgettable phone call had signaled the beginning of our transplant journey. My first day back at work confirmed that my life was moving forward; I was home.

Growth is the only evidence of life.
—John Henry Newman

Lifting the Veil

Our lives continued to move forward, and Doug's Prednisone haze slowly and progressively lifted. As the haze cleared, I was thrilled to discover that I had a new and improved version of my old husband. Doug's smile slowly returned, and the old sparkle in his eyes returned and shone with a renewed vigor. His personality softened, tears and emotion came more easily, and he spoke daily of his love and gratitude for my presence in his life. It was not unusual for him to just sit and stare at me as if I were a brilliant piece of art in the Louvre.

I was initially uncomfortable with all of the attention that he lavished upon me, but as time passed, I grew quite fond of the flattery. His willingness to be so expressive and open created an avenue for extremely deep conversations, and for the first time in our marriage, we felt completely free to unleash all of our fears, emotions, and guilt.

After we were married, we would engage in academic conversations about religion and the meaning of life, but the comfort and routine of marriage made it easy to skirt real emotion. As a result, we developed an unhealthy habit of locking away our deepest thoughts and fears in an attempt to protect ourselves and one another. We had walked in the shadow of death for so long that it became easier to just push away the emotions that gnawed relentlessly at our hearts. Talking hurt, and we had enough hurt in our lives. In fact, our very survival became dependent upon a certain level of denial and unspoken fear. We cried together whenever the doctor would give us bad news, and we would discuss and research medical options endlessly, but we did our best to avoid the real and true articulation of our feelings.

At a most basic level, our feelings could be summarized in one sentence: I feared Doug's death, and he feared abandoning and hurting me. These feelings were certainly intense enough, but they were also compounded by tremendous feelings of guilt. Doug felt guilty that our lives were so often disrupted by his illness, and as his disease progressed, he felt guilty that he was able to do less and less, and I had to do more and more. I felt guilty because I would also get angry that our lives were so limited by his disease and that I was always the one who had to pick up the extra slack and miss work.

I hated sitting in doctors' offices, hospitals, and waiting rooms. I hated waiting for the results of a test or hearing a doctor's grim news. I hated the way family and friends viewed me as the wonderful and patient caregiver. I didn't feel the way people saw me. How could I? My heart ached, and I lived in a world of constant uncertainty. I wasn't patient or wonderful. I was scared and angry. I hated the constant question, "How's Doug doing?" But most of all, I hated watching Doug suffer and struggle. I hated the pale pallor that signaled illness, I hated the crackling sound of his lungs, and I hated the look of fear and weariness that he often donned after a doctor's visit. I was helpless to change the course of his disease, and I hated that fact.

My feelings of anger and resentment repulsed me, and I was caught in a vicious circle of anger and guilt. I would get angry about my circumstances and then feel guilty about being angry. My Catholic background had taught me to feel guilty about everything, and I knew that the nuns and priests of my past would be quite impressed and pleased with their work. They had taught me well.

I should have shared all of this with Doug, but I didn't want to hurt him or compound the guilt that I knew he already felt. Instead, I chose to release my emotions by crying alone in the shower. It was therapeutic and cleansing, and I viewed my time in the shower as an extremely healthy therapy. By George, I was dealing with my feelings. I was an idiot.

My feelings stayed locked in a box in my mind, and I was unwilling to share them with anyone. Al Gore may want to take credit for the "lockbox" concept, but it was really my creation. I could not control Doug's health, but I could control how I dealt with my emotions. Unfortunately, I chose to control my emotions by hiding them. They were mine, and they would stay that way. One way or another, I was going to control some part of my life.

Conversely, Doug distanced himself emotionally from me in an attempt to ease the constant guilt and fear that he felt. He avoided or minimized discussions about any feelings and fears that were related to his health. I would push him to talk about what he was feeling, but the topics were just too painful, and he would erect a brick wall that I was either unwilling or unable to scale.

I was often frustrated by his unwillingness to talk about his health, but I was a hypocrite. I wanted to know what he was feeling, and it angered me when he wouldn't talk. I wanted and expected him to be the one who would break the emotional ice. There were many times that I wanted to grab him and tell him that he was full of crap. "I know that you're scared. Tell me what you're feeling." But I wasn't even honest enough to challenge him. I was just as scared and incapable of being real as he was. In an attempt to avoid hurting one another, we stagnated the growth of our relationship by unnecessarily isolating ourselves and needlessly dancing alone to the tune of our unspoken fears.

What we didn't realize prior to Doug's transplant was that our inability to venture into the pain, guilt, and emptiness that pervaded our world only intensified the anguish. It was so easy to sweep the hurt under the rug, avoid conversations, or suffer alone in a shower. It was easy to stay in a place where we were nice and polite and avoided the emotional landmines. But as a result, we missed so many opportunities to deepen our relationship. We needed to embrace the difficult emotions that engulfed us if we were ever going to move beyond the pain to grow and become open and honest partners united in our battle against the unruly child.

The transplant experience finally allowed us to get real with one another. We had met Dante and toured his proverbial Inferno repeatedly. We were emotionally raw, and there was simply nothing left to hide. Every emotion had been experienced, but what still remained elusive was complete emotional honesty. To achieve this honesty, we had to start by revealing our deepest emotions and allowing ourselves to be completely vulnerable in the other's presence. We began to affectionately refer to this process as having an emotional enema.

Doug was the first one who dared to break through the emotional barrier that we had erected, and I gladly followed his lead. His new openness began while he was still hospitalized. He had been fully conscious for just a few days when he decided to tell me that he would never consider having an affair with another woman. I was a little confused by his words because they literally came out of nowhere. We had just finished a conversation about hospital food when he suddenly jumped to the topic of extramarital affairs. I blamed the bizarre topic change on his medication, and while the meds did play a large part, Doug was a changed man, and he was willing to talk about any emotions or thoughts that crossed the synapses of his mind.

He began by telling me that all men have urges. Oh dear Lord! Where is this conversation going? I sheepishly wondered.

"Yes, Doug. Men do seem to have urges," I countered.

"Well Dana, I have urges too, and there are a lot of really pretty girls I'd love to sleep with. But I never would do it because I have the best wife in the world, and I would never do anything to hurt you or jeopardize what we have. I love you more than anything in the world."

I think that I was touched by his words, but I could not seem to get past his declaration that there were a lot of pretty girls that he would just love to sleep with. I initially didn't know how to respond, so I just smiled and nodded at him. "Well, that's very good to know, Doug," I eventually managed to say through my laughter. He smiled contentedly, and it was obvious that he was quite pleased with his profound revelation and proclamation of supreme devotion to me.

Doug continued to reveal things to me that I never knew he felt. He would often engage in these conversations as soon as I would come home from work. He had been alone with his thoughts for nine hours, and he couldn't wait to share them with me. So the minute I would step in the door, he would start a deep conversation. I was always thrilled at the prospect of having a meaningful conversation, but there were several days in which I couldn't help thinking that I could have used an hour or two of decompression time before engaging in such profound conversations. I had just spent several hours with over one hundred goofy teenagers, and it was hard to immediately switch gears and have a deeply adult conversation.

Among many things, Doug revealed to me that he had always pictured himself dying alone in a hospital or in his sister's house. Through tears, he told me that he could have never imagined being lucky enough to find a girl like me who could love him and support him the way that I had. I was deeply touched, and I was grateful that the transplant had given us this moment. At that instant, I thought that if everything were to end tomorrow, the moment I had just shared with him made every struggle, frustration, and tear worth it.

Doug also revealed to me that he worried incessantly about what I would do if he died. Wow, emotional vulnerability was what I had always wanted, but this vulnerability stuff was tougher than I had imagined. After stammering for a bit, I told him that while I do fear his death, I do my best not to dwell on it. It is such a perverse waste of time. While I am stewing about his death, I'm neglecting the fact that he is alive and in my life.

I also turned the tables on him, and I asked him what he would do if I died tomorrow. He looked stunned, as if the thought had never even crossed his mind. I reminded him that I too was mortal and that just because I don't have a disease does not guarantee me tomorrow. We are all living on borrowed time, my friend. The old adage that we should savor each day as our last is good advice for the healthy and the sick. Having a chronic or terminal illness just gives an individual and his or her family the advantage of truly understanding the meaning and importance of those words. In addition, anyone who is willing to open his or her heart to love has to be open to the possibility of loss. Someone has to die first, and someone has to be left behind. It's just the way life is.

Doug also asked me if I would remarry again if he were to die first. He then told me that he wanted me to remarry because he wanted me to be happy. I was caught off guard by the question, and the cool emotional façade that I had worn during the "What will you do when I'm dead?" conversation crumbled, and the tears began to flow. I didn't know what to say; I wanted to revert to my comfort zone. I wanted to bottle my emotions and move on to another topic. This hurt too much. Where was my shower?

I told him that I didn't know the answer to his question, but what I did know was that we were both alive, and we had a new lease on life. You are still here, and you are my husband. That's enough for today, and if we are lucky enough to be blessed with another day of life, it will be enough for tomorrow. Some people spend a lifetime seeking their purpose, but I was blessed to know my purpose. I was Doug's companion in sickness and in health, and together we were blessed to experience and learn the lessons of a chronic illness and a renewed life.

As time progressed, we continued to talk, and we released virtually every fear and emotion that had been stifled and catalogued over the years. The process was extremely cathartic, and we came to the conclusion that our feelings were neither right nor wrong; they just were. We were entitled to feel whatever we felt, but we were now obligated to be open and honest with one another. Doug had new lungs and a new lease on life, and we were going to make the most out of it.

Being honest and open allowed us to turn our pain into relational growth, and our love quickly deepened. We discovered that we had to immerse ourselves in the pain if we ever hoped to be free from the pain. The shadows that once lived in our emotional closets were no longer hidden. It was as if we had been living in Plato's cave. We had been bound to the fear of the shadows, but once we revealed the truth to one another, we came out of the cave and basked in the freedom of the light.

Friends are those rare people who ask how we are and then wait to hear the answer.

—Ed Cunningham

Lessons in a Waiting Room

There are many lessons to be learned in a hospital, and the waiting room became one of my many classrooms. But this time, the tables had been turned. I was no longer the teacher; I was now the student who was force-fed daily lessons. My first lesson was short and simple, and my understanding of the concept was complete and immediate: a hospital waiting room offers very little in the way of physical comfort.

When the waiting room became my new home, my first goal was to find a comfortable spot in which I could relax while waiting for my short and sporadic visits with Doug. This was a daunting challenge, and I eventually had to accept the fact that physical comfort just could not be found.

I tried every chair and every couch within a short radius of Doug's wing, and I even attempted multiple positions in various chairs. I was never a gymnast, but I am quite certain that some of the routines that I performed in the chairs while attempting to find a comfortable position would have rivaled that of an Olympic champion. I know that I would have lost points for grace, choreography, and the all-important dismount, but my chair routines would have certainly scored big points for improvisational creativity and effort.

There were, however, two rocking chairs in the waiting room that were extremely comfortable, and their comfort was enhanced by the smooth rocking motion that helped to soothe and calm the persistent anxiety that pervaded the area. But it did not take long for people to discover this fact, and the chairs became very hot commodities. Once an individual achieved the glory of securing the rocking chair, it was always a difficult and gut wrenching choice to relinquish it. Every time a nurse would beckon me to Doug's room, my mind would silently and sarcastically say, "Doug wants to see me now? Does he realize that I just got the rocking chair?"

In addition to the lack of physical comfort, there were also few creature comforts. The magazines were old and bad, and the artwork was even worse. The coffee from the vending machine tasted like weak battery acid, and it was comical to watch the same people buy the same evil coffee repeatedly each morning in the hope that it just might have improved overnight. But each sip would inevitability result in the same puckered and disappointed face. Hope springs eternal in a hospital, and that same hope endured in every coffee drinker's belief that one special day the coffee machine just might produce a succulent cup of coffee.

The food from the vending machines was no better than the coffee. There was plenty of sodium, sugar, and fat to make any coronary artery quiver in fear, and most of the offerings could have only been appetizing to someone who had grown weary of coconuts and bananas after being marooned for years on a desert island.

In our boredom, my brother and I would occasionally stand in front of the vending machine and push the button that would make the food carrousel rotate. It was often more entertaining than watching television, and we were often amazed to discover that the food in the hospital cafeteria was just a hot version of the vending machine crap that rotated in front of our faces.

They say some animals will eat their own kind in times of desperation, and I knew that I had reached a new low when I started visualizing doctors as walking bowls of al dente pasta covered in a simple and surprisingly zesty marinara sauce. I wasn't sure if the visions represented repressed anger or a deep and persistent craving for edible food.

My second lesson was more complex and profound, and its meaning and magnitude slowly evolved over time. This lesson was not about a simple understanding of physical comfort, but it was a lesson of emotional comfort. Hidden among the uncomfortable furniture, the bad coffee, and the steady stream of activity, I learned that there were rich blessings to be found in the faces and words of the human beings who had also been thrown unwittingly into the hospital classroom known as the waiting room.

The consistent presence of my family and friends in the waiting room brought me tremendous comfort. We vacillated between conversation and watching television, and we even made a few feeble attempts at reading. But we soon discovered that reading was virtually impossible, as our overwhelmed psyches lacked the necessary focus, and we began to feel like we had suddenly been stricken with severe cases of attention deficit disorder. In addition, the constant rumbling of squeaky food carts, wheelchairs, gurneys, and portable x-ray machines provided a constant source of distraction that made it virtually impossible to concentrate.

My brother finally decided to buy a stack of mindless celebrity and tabloid magazines that required virtually no cerebral acuity. We had regressed to a childhood state in which we only wanted pictures—no words, thank you very much. The magazines were a huge hit, and people who would have never been caught dead with a National Enquirer were suddenly willing to savor its idiocy in an attempt to pass the time.

We also found reason to laugh from time to time. I love to laugh, and I was elated by anything that provided an opportunity to temporarily escape from my fear and worry. My brother was my biggest source of laughter, as he and I share the same sense of humor. Even in our darkest hours, we were always able to find something to giggle about through our tears. As Dolly Parton said in the movie *Steel Magnolias,* "Laughter through tears is my favorite emotion." Ugh, shut up Dolly!

Doug had always been perplexed by the fact that my brother and I always had the ability to laugh and carry on even at the most inappropriate times, and it made me happy to know that Doug would have been shaking his head at us as we laughed our way through the difficult process. There was a normalcy in our laughter and in my vision of Doug's response to it, and I found tremendous comfort in that.

My dad was also present and became my companion as everyone else came and went. He was my one and constant presence in the waiting room, and he would keep me company from morning till night. And whenever I spent time alone with Doug, he waited patiently for hours. He never complained, and he somehow managed to keep himself amused and entertained in the pits of boredom.

I was never more thankful for my father than when I would come out to the waiting room after spending hours engaged in my nightly routine of soothing Doug in an attempt to help him fall asleep. It could be eleven o'clock at night, and there would be my father waiting patiently for me. He frequently looked tired, but his patience would never wane. He would snap to attention and ask me the same question, "How's he doing tonight?" That was always my cue to spill whatever emotion I wanted to release, and my father would always listen to whatever I was willing to share with him.

We would then bid a fond adieu to the waiting room and begin our walk back to the hotel. We always knew that our time in the hotel would be short because the waiting room would once again beckon us early the next morning. I could not have endured the transplant experience and the waiting room without my father. He and I endured countless hours in the waiting room, and his presence was calming and helped me to maintain a sense of balance, harmony, and sanity.

My mother lived out of state and was unable to come to Wisconsin because of her health. But despite the fact that she was not physically present, I knew that her spirit was with me in that waiting room. I wanted her there desperately, but my father, brother, and I had a unique opportunity to spend more time together than we ever had before.

My father had traveled a great deal when we were children, so my brother and I spent most of our time with our mother. Doug's transplant gave us the perfect opportunity to make up for lost time, and the three of us were finally able to share an unparalleled barrage of joy and sadness. Doug's transplant was agonizingly difficult for all of us, but it was a tremendous blessing that allowed my brother and me to renew and strengthen our bond with our father. Once again, beauty and understanding had arisen from that which was dark and difficult.

The waiting room was not only filled with my family and friends, but it was also filled with two families who were engaged in the same lung transplant journey. One man had received his transplant due to Emphysema, while the other man had received his due to cystic fibrosis. Both families had been on the journey longer than I, and I was grateful for their guidance as the new kid on the transplant block. There is always an amazing and instant bond that is forged between individuals who are enduring the same process and struggle, and I immediately felt a connection to the two families.

Each day, as we would arrive at the hospital, we greeted one another with what quickly became our standard question: "How are things?" We would give the latest details on everything that had occurred, and we would inevitably swap doctor, nurse, and treatment stories.

Over time, I learned to read the faces of the other families, and their joy and pain was clearly evident even before I had an opportunity to ask how things were. The weariness that we wore on our faces and the sadness and worry that veiled our eyes became our common bond. We celebrated and rejoiced in the progress that our boys made, and we grieved each setback as if it had occurred to a member of our own family. We were a support group for one another, and we began to rely on one another's presence.

I cannot imagine having gone through this experience without the guidance and support of the two other transplant families and my own family and friends. I truly believe that God placed the three families together in Madison at the same time so that we could support and sustain one another. We are not intended to be alone in darkness, and

God sent me a beacon of light by blessing me with the presence of my own family and friends and the two wonderful families who endured the process with us.

For wisdom is far more valuable than rubies. Nothing you desire can be compared with it.

—Proverbs 8:11 (NLT)

Reflections of the Past

"He has cystic fibrosis, and he'll be lucky to live to the age of seven." The fifteen words that cascaded from the doctor's mouth were arranged in such a manner that their reality would forever alter the life of anyone who dared to love a man named Doug Broehl. But while the reality of Doug's diagnosis was full of heartache, entwined within the heartache were lessons in character, perseverance, determination, and love. Illness alters people's lives irrevocably, but the journey is eased by companionship, and the results of the shared struggle can result in a new and invigorating life vision.

Doug's diagnosis permanently altered the lives of his parents. Life as they once knew it ended with his diagnosis. Their young son had received a death sentence, and they were left to cope with a world that was assailed by fear, uncertainty, anger, and a constant state of vulnerability. Doug's parents could have easily made a decision to immerse themselves in a world of self-pity, but they chose to fight the illness and treat their son as a normal child, for indeed he was a normal child who just happened to have an illness.

Early in our marriage, Doug's mother had shared a story with me that reflected her determination and commitment to giving Doug a normal childhood. Each day she, his father, or his sister would spend thirty minutes twice a day clapping Doug's chest and back in an attempt to loosen the secretions in his lungs. Doug hated the sessions, and he would do everything in his power to avoid them. He was occasionally given a reprieve on his birthday, but chest therapy was normally a non-negotiable issue in the Broehl house. However, after his therapy session was completed, Doug was free to go, play, and do as he pleased.

On one particularly cold and snowy day, Doug headed outside to play after his morning chest therapy. A neighbor across the street, who was perhaps a little overly vigilant in her neighborly duties, called to inform Doug's mom that her little sick convict had escaped and was playing outside in the cold. Doug's mom calmly told the neighbor that she already knew that he was playing outside.

"I cannot believe that you spend all that time on his therapy, and then you just squander it by letting him play in the cold," said the dumbfounded neighbor.

Doug's mom quickly retorted, "He's a normal boy who just wants to play outside. I am not going to let his illness stop him from doing what every other boy in the neighborhood is doing."

And so it was with that resolve that Doug's parents gave him the opportunity to be just another normal little boy on the block.

As the years past, their baby boy grew up to do many of the things that all parents envision for their children. Doug graduated from high school and college, traveled through Europe, taught at a university, wrote a dissertation, got married, honeymooned in Cancun, bought a house, and began to gray around the temples. He was living the American dream in spite of a serious illness, and he was discovering that happiness and fulfillment were not reserved only for the healthy and able bodied. Doug was a survivor, and he would not die at the age of seven as his doctors had predicted. Through a little genetic luck and a mountain of determination, he would survive into adulthood. Cystic fibrosis does kill children, but it would not kill this child. Doug had defied the odds, and his life would not be reduced to a statistic.

Despite his survival into adulthood, his disease would continue to progress, and it would eventually claim his lungs. At thirty-eight years of age, Doug was dying, and the disease was doing its best to claim him. He was losing the battle, and that fact was officially confirmed on the day he was listed for a transplant. The possibility of death and the sting of the label end-stage cystic fibrosis loomed heavily in our lives, but the possibility of a transplant and a new and transformed life lessened the sting. We would not give up hope.

Just as Doug's parents had refused to relinquish their child to this disease, so we too would do everything in our power to refuse to bow to its fate. We were terrified, but we were more committed than ever to each other and our battle against his illness. Doug would survive the wait for a transplant, and although he was able to elude the death grip of his disease, his challenges would not end. He had traded one disease for another, and he would continue to have a daily battle for his life. But his transplant rekindled the hope of a new life, and that hope shone brilliantly.

The battles against cystic fibrosis and the physical and emotional battles of his transplant were grueling, but the lessons we learned about living and loving in the shadow of an illness were worth every tear and every ounce of pain. But despite the wisdom we have gained, our journey is not complete; there is still much more ahead for us. And we know that no matter what the future has in store for us, we will weather the experience together and continue to grow and learn from life and each other.

No one should journey through an illness alone; illness requires companionship. The journey through an illness is made easier when we allow ourselves to be loved and when we allow ourselves to be vulnerable in another's presence. God calls us to love and seek companionship in our lives, and that call is never more critical than in times of illness.

Relationships provide us with the greatest opportunities to grow, learn, love, and be wounded, and when the relationship is with someone who is ill, the opportunities for growth and heartache are intensified. As a result, the relationship will either be strengthened or broken. If we can persevere through the challenges and the heartache, we can learn who we truly are and what truly matters in our lives. The unexamined life is pointless, and the unchallenged life provides little opportunity for personal growth. Illness requires a commitment and a determination, and it provides a call to love and trust in what life gives to us.

At the end of the road, whether the end of a struggle is happy or sad, illness strips the insignificant from our lives, and we are left with the realization that each moment in life is a precious gift that is meant to be savored. Our priorities change, our facades fall, and the search and the need for meaning become the focus of our existence. Illness is a battle that challenges our character and requires us to back up our beliefs; illness demands that we back our words, vows, and commitments with our actions.

On our wedding day, Doug and I exchanged vows, and we made a deep and solemn commitment to one another. Philosophers and theologians have searched endlessly for the meaning of life, but it is really so very simple. We are called to love, and we are called to endure no matter what the circumstances. I thought that I understood the meaning of the vows that I spoke to him on that chilly October day, but what I didn't realize was that the meaning of life is found in a one line sentence that is uttered at virtually every wedding: "I take you, to be my husband/wife, and I promise before God and these witnesses to be your loving and faithful husband/wife, for richer, for poorer, in joy and sorrow, in sickness and health, as long as we both shall live."

So don't worry about tomorrow, for tomorrow will bring its own worries. Today's trouble is enough for today.

—Matthew 6:34 (NLT)

Day by Day: A Transplant Journal

I wrote the following emails to family, friends, and our two online support groups during the course of Doug's transplant. My initial intention was to provide a brief medical update on a daily basis. But as time progressed, and I began to feel the full impact of the experience, my emails grew in length and became more reflective, introspective, and emotionally raw.

What began as a simple means of providing brief updates turned into a cathartic journal of my experiences. I wrote the majority of the emails at night after spending the day at the hospital. Reflecting upon the day helped me to process and purge my emotions before I would begin the often futile process of trying to sleep. The opportunity to write about and reflect upon each day was extremely therapeutic, and having the chance to express my thoughts and emotions to an audience of people who cared about Doug helped me endure the sometimes overwhelming challenges of the experience.

The emails are also occasionally critical of the hospital in which Doug had his transplant. I stand by this criticism, but at the same time, I would highly recommend University Hospital to anyone who is considering a transplant. It is an imperfect place, as is any hospital or institution. But UW Madison is also a hospital that is full of some of the best and brightest doctors in the world. The transplant surgeon is a gifted and skilled man who has a tremendously successful track record, and the nurses on the transplant unit are simply phenomenal. We are eternally grateful to all of the doctors and nurses who cared for Doug at UW, and there is simply no way that we can ever truly express our gratitude for our second chance at life.

4/01/03

After only a five month wait, Doug received his new lungs on Monday evening. He came through the surgery very well, but had a bit of a setback on Tuesday afternoon. His new lungs are swollen and have been traumatized by the surgery, so they are struggling to keep him oxygenated. To give his new lungs a rest, the doctors have put him on a machine that oxygenates his blood and turned down the ventilator. The hope is that this will allow his lungs to heal so that they can then handle the load. Beyond this, his other organs are performing perfectly, and he seems to be very peaceful. There are no words that can describe how difficult it is to see him like this. I am so desperate for this to work. On the way to the hospital, his main concern was for me. He just kept saying that he wanted this to work for me, and I'm sitting next to him thinking, "I just want this to work for you." He deserves this second chance so much. I'm currently using my brother's computer, but a friend of mine is bringing mine up tomorrow, so I will be able to send out updates as time permits. Please keep him in your prayers, and if you don't mind, say a prayer or two for me. I've never felt so emotionally raw, and I sometimes wonder how I'll make it through this.

4/02/03

Doug continues to be stable. His vital signs are perfect, and his other organs are performing perfectly. If he continues to do well, they will begin weaning him from the ECMO machine within the next twenty-four hours. The ECMO is the machine that oxygenates his blood so that his lungs can heal. He looked great today. His cheeks were rosy, and he looked very peaceful. The doctor told me that things are going very well and that his chest x-rays continue to look great. As always, I am overwhelmed by the kindness and sweetness that people have shown to me. I normally make it a point to respond to every email that I receive, but I am going to beg for a little indulgence this time. So for everyone who sent me a note, I offer you a collective and heartfelt THANK YOU! For those of you who inquired, I will send a room number for cards when that becomes available. Thank you again for your kind words and your thoughts and prayers, and I will do my best to keep you updated. Now go and pray for us!

4/03/03

Today was a good day for Doug. They were able to wean him off of the ECMO machine which was giving his lungs an opportunity to heal. His lungs are now functioning and are keeping him well oxygenated with the aid of the ventilator. They will continue to monitor him closely, and if things remain stable, they will start to wake him in the next few days. He still looks good, and he is still very peaceful. I can't wait to see his eyes again, and I can't wait to talk to him—I miss him terribly. Please continue your thoughts and prayers for him.

4/04/03

Doug had another great day today. They began to wean him from the vent, and they woke him up. His vent was set at 95 percent yesterday, and it is currently at 64 percent. The doctors are very pleased with his progress and are very optimistic. I was able to speak to him today, and he is able to respond to yes or no questions. Unfortunately, when he is awake, he is very uncomfortable, and he hates the vent tube. The nurse asked him if he wanted more sedation, which resulted in a very hardy head nod. It breaks my heart to see him uncomfortable, but it was wonderful to see his eyes and be able to talk to him. Please keep those prayers coming. For those of you who have expressed concerns about my not eating and not sleeping issues, I actually ate three meals today, and my brother talked me into taking a Valium last night. Yes, better sleeping is possible through a little chemistry experiment.

4/05/03

Things continue to go smoothly. The doctors began to wean him from the NO2 machine (don't ask, my mind is too tired to explain), and they have the ventilator as low as it can go. When the NO2 machine is turned off, they will then begin the process of weaning him from the ventilator. When that happens, I will begin weaning myself from the multitude of pharmaceuticals and narcotics—that's a joke. Do I hear any laughter? Work with me people, I need your pity. Anyway, Doug's vitals were great today. His blood pressure is beautiful, his pulse is perfect, his oxygen saturation is running between 96-97 percent, and the doctor told me that he is doing very well. His kidneys are being a bit fussy, but the doctor said that it is nothing terrible and that it is par for the course in transplantation. He was conscious again today, and I was able to talk to him quite a bit. I did discover that we are not good at charades. My brain is mush, and I'm supposed to be intuitive and insightful? He continues to be agitated by the vent, and they have tied his hands down to keep him from removing it. I spent a lot of time scratching his itches—he is going to owe me big time for this! He also likes to have just about every part of his body massaged, as it seems to soothe him. He reminded me of a dog today because every time I hit a spot that he really liked, his head went up and down like a fiend. Well, that's about all. Thank you for all of your support, your kind words, and your prayers.

4/06/03

The progress continues to be positive. Doug was very alert today, and we were able to play a long game of charades again. It was a bit of a challenge, and let's just say that when I told Doug that he needed to marry a smarter woman in his next life, he didn't disagree. The doctor continues to be pleased with his progress, and he is looking to remove his vent tube by Tuesday. Again, I would like to thank everyone for their kind words and thoughts. I started to tell Doug about all of the support that family and friends have given, but it was just too emotionally difficult for him today. I'm fairly certain that after the vent is removed, the two of us are just going to sit, cry, and thank God for every tear of joy and relief.

4/07/03

Doug had another very good day, and I HATE charades with the passion of 10,000 blazing suns. The poor man must have rolled his eyes at me a thousand times. I truly think that he has resigned himself to the fact that he has indeed married the village idiot. The nitric oxide machine has been turned off, and they are going to let him have a good rest tonight. Tomorrow is the big day for weaning from the vent, so I'm excited and scared. So hey pilgrims, can we rustle up some prayers for cowboy Doug? I don't know why I just called him a cowboy, but it just seemed to flow with rustling and pilgrims. I must find a way to get some sleep.

4/08/03

Children, today we will be learning about a little thing called FRUSTRATION. Doug is still doing very well, but he is becoming more active and "talkative" everyday. This is a wonderful thing, but he won't be quiet, and half of the time I don't know what in the HELL he is trying to say. I'm sorry children, Mrs. Broehl wants to swear like a sailor right now. This afternoon, in a state of exhaustion and frustration, I told him that I couldn't do it anymore. I updated him on his health, told him about every family member and friend who has ever existed in his life, and then begged a nurse to sedate him. Now before you think that Doug has married the Antichrist, the nurse agreed that he was expending way too much energy, and so she helped him take a little chemical nap. Also, they did try to wean him from the vent, but it did not go well. He became very anxious, and he said that his chest hurt too much. The doctors and nurses said that this is a very common occurrence and that they will try again tomorrow. The doctor's statement was, "Don't worry, we'll get there." Okay doctor, can Dana have a chemical nap, and can you wake her when we get there?

4/09/03

Well, it happened today. The vent was finally removed this afternoon, and Doug's lungs are functioning perfectly. It was, without a doubt, the most emotional moment of my life. I was there when they pulled out the tube, and I heard the first "gasp" of his new lungs. We immediately put them to the test by having a good long cry. Doug is currently experiencing some anxiety because of sleep deprivation, drugs, and an inability to comprehend the ability to breathe again. But he is working through it. He needed assurance on a fairly regular basis, and he wanted to talk or have someone talk to him constantly. On one occasion, while trying to maintain a constant stream of conversation, I told him that people were dancing in the streets of Baghdad. In his confusion, he asked me if they were celebrating transplants! Yes, there's a party in Baghdad for Doug's new lungs. By the way, thank you to everyone who has sent a card to us. I tried to read some of them to Doug today, but he had the attention span of a mosquito. You don't like or understand the analogy? Watch the little bloodsuckers this summer just jumping aimlessly from person to person, and you'll understand what I'm talking about. I hear all of you: "She's babbling, she's still not sleeping; she's delirious." Leave me alone people, I've got to get to the transplant party in Baghdad.

4/10/03

Doug continues to do well, but he is extremely anxious. He needed assurance just about every five minutes today. He has been rambling for two days about Dante's Inferno, the pits of hell, and doctors with flaming hair and eyes. In the late afternoon, two doctors and a group of med students came in to see him, and he had a minor anxiety attack. The five white coats scared him, and for some reason, he thought that they had come in to take his dinner tray. They assured him that they had no intention of taking his food, and I reminded him that Madison is a teaching hospital with doctors who travel in packs—like wolves. That was probably a bad analogy for a guy who is so easily scared now. Yes Doug, there are five wolves in your room, and I just saw Dante, and he's stoking the fires of hell as we speak. Anyway, he had two of his chest tubes removed, walked in place for a few minutes, and ate his first meal today. As I was leaving this evening, and after using my best Tony Robbins' positive affirmation lines to bolster his confidence, Doug told me that it was a very good day and that tomorrow would be even better. That's right, Doug. Hey Dante, lay down that fiery pitchfork and stay the HELL away from us.

4/11/03

I tried to send an update last night, but my typing was too slurred. Stop. Reread that line again because it is slightly amusing. Doug had a superb day yesterday. The confusion, delirium, hallucinations, and anxiety finally began to wane, and the Doug we all know and love came back to life. He was finally able to understand and savor the fact that he is alive and doing very well. He was also able to walk down the hall, and it was an amazing triumph for him. It's amazing to see him grow physically stronger everyday, and it's amazing to be around him and not hear coughing and crackling lungs. Whenever we would go to a store and go our separate ways, I always used his cough as a tracking device to find him. I told him that I didn't know how I was going to be able to find him anymore, but then I remembered that my uterus also doubles as a tracking device. But I'll have to really concentrate because the uterine signal sometimes gets blocked in the bigger stores. Before I wrap this up, I again wanted to thank everyone who has shown us so much kindness and support. I have been receiving over forty emails and four to five cards a day, and I savor and appreciate every single one of them. I would love to respond to each and every one of them, but that darn Doug just keeps monopolizing my time. I'm just about ready to tell him to hop off of this little attention getting gravy train. Honestly, such a little ego maniac—me, me, me! Okay, I'll stop with the sarcasm and end this on a very serious and heartfelt note. I really can't recommend this experience to anyone, but it has truly been the most profound and life altering experience of my life, and I thank God that he has given me the strength and support to endure. So in Doug's honor today, go outside, take a deep breath, count your blessings, and savor the incredible beauty of life.

4/12/03

I received quite a few emails asking about how I am able to use my uterus as a tracking device. I must come clean now and admit that my uterus does not have superpowers. Since the standard joke is that all men think with their unmentionable, I decided long ago that I wanted a second brain too. So I started joking that my uterus could track airplanes, boats, surface to air missiles, Santa Claus, and Doug. I likened it to having my own personal GPS system. So relax men, the uterus can't really track you.

Doug had another very good day, but he was quite sleepy. He has been ungodly chatty ever since they removed the vent, and yesterday was no different. It was a bit comical to watch him yesterday because he would just be jabbering and then fall asleep mid-sentence. He was still a bit goofy yesterday, but he is now very cognizant of his goofy moments. When he was sleeping yesterday, he suddenly opened his eyes and said, "You know Dana, the world is a very fragile place." He then fell asleep again only to pop up a few minutes later with, "Glass bulbs are fragile too." He then looked at me, laughed, and said, "I have no idea why I just said that!" On the medical side, he had all of his IV and arterial lines removed, and he now has only one central line. We just have to wait now for the last two chest tubes to be removed, and he will then be virtually tubeless and cordless. He also did his first lung function test yesterday. His first numbers were significantly higher than his old lung numbers, but they were not as high as I had hoped that they would be. But when they did the same test again six hours later, his numbers jumped forty points. I haven't talked to any doctors about this, so I'm assuming that these numbers will continue to rise as he heals and gets stronger. The best news is that he was released from the ICU. Unfortunately, there were no empty rooms on the regular wing. We are hoping that he will have a new room today, and I'll send an address when I receive one. Thanks again for all of your kind words and support.

4/13/03

It was another good day for Doug. I know that line sounds like a skipping record, but don't touch it—I'll hurt you. Doug was able to walk faster and further today, and he is now able to get himself in and out of bed with virtually no assistance. He is counting the days until he can put on underwear and pajama pants. I'm also counting the days, as he has flashed me too many times. It would be exciting if we were at home, but it just loses something in a hospital room. Eww, that was probably too much information. Anyway, we are still waiting for a regular room, and he is hoping to get his remaining chest tubes removed today. The highlight of yesterday was going outside with him. We were able to take him to a fourth floor observatory and spend fifteen minutes soaking up the sun and the warm temperatures. It was such a simple thing that we all take for granted, but it was a big moment. To be able to be outside with Doug again, feel the sun on my face, and be able to look over a city filled with life reminded me of just how lucky and blessed we truly are. So haul your collective asses outside again and savor life.

4/14/03

Did everyone have a chance to haul ass yesterday? I hope so, because Doug and I hauled our collective derrieres all over the place. A room on the regular wing finally opened, and Doug was set free. We burst through the doors of the ICU and ran down the halls singing, "The hills are alive with the sound of music." Okay, that's a lie, but it was wonderful to be set free. My brother and I were able to take him to the cafeteria, down to the lounge, and outside. Don't worry, he had his mask on, and we had permission from his doctors. It was superb for Doug to see something new. He also had his chest tubes removed yesterday, and it was a very good thing because he was becoming extremely cranky about them. Today they will do a biopsy of his lungs to see if there are any signs of rejection, and we will have the results on Wednesday. I'm a little nervous about this, but nervous has become my new state of being. If things go well, they will begin teaching him about his new meds, and they said that he could be released in a week or so. I try not to think that far down the line because I have discovered that it's best to take things one day at a time. I would again appreciate your prayers and thoughts for him as he has his biopsy today.

4/15/03

Doug had his bronchoscopy today, and he was very irritated by the fact that it made him loopy again. Thankfully, he was a quiet loopy. But not to worry, once he came out of the fog, he walked and talked like a madman. We walked up to the observatory, and we were able to sit outside again. He told me that he used to sit there when he was hospitalized for IV's as a teenager. He said that he could have never imagined then that someday he would get married and have a second chance at life because of a transplant. It is just so incredible to see him so happy and walking and breathing with such ease. He also had his best numbers yet on his breathing test today. I just can't tell you how elated he is. We will get the results of the bronchoscopy tomorrow, and I will then be able to start breathing again. Doug is a lovely shade of pink, and I'm turning blue. We would make great bookends in a baby's room. See you tomorrow, my people.

4/16/03

Today was an extremely trying day, but I will begin with the best news of the day: Doug's biopsy showed absolutely no signs of rejection! I arrived early this morning to be greeted by a slightly overzealous nurse who virtually body blocked me from entering the room. I could have taken her, but I don't like to release my superpowers in public. Anyway, she informed me that I would have to wear a gown, gloves, and a mask because Doug had been placed in isolation due to a positive culture of Pseudomonas and Aspergillus from his bronch yesterday. After donning my nuclear waste suit of armor, I asked Doug what in the world was going on. Unfortunately, he knew no more than I did, so we decided to call in his nurse in an attempt to get some answers. His nurse told him that he didn't culture those things in his bronch, but it was a possibility that he might in the future. I might get cancer in the future. Should we start chemotherapy today or tomorrow? We then had the nurse page his transplant coordinator, and when she came up to see us, she said, "Why are you in isolation?" Well, Groucho Marx, that's the secret question of the day! We also complained about the fact that since Doug moved from the ICU, not one of his transplant doctors had been by to examine or talk to him. She seemed a bit appalled and left on a mission to solve the mysteries. Amazingly enough, after a very short while, Doug was removed from isolation, and two doctors paid him a visit—lousy sewer rat bastards—oops, pardon my French. The bottom line is this: there are no signs of rejection, the cultures have come back clean, and his new lungs look good. They are going to perform another bronch on Monday to check an area where the lung was connected to Doug's old hardware. It's healing slowly, and they want to monitor it to make sure that there is no dead tissue that could lead to infection. If things go well, they are talking about releasing him early next week. So the news was very good today, but we were extremely annoyed by the other events of the day. We are both discovering that our patience is waning. When Doug took a walk today, we were dancing around his closet (AKA hospital room) trying to get everything situated. "My pants are slipping, I need that cord moved, move that walker toward me, grab that portable oxygen tank, etc., etc." I was just exhausted, and I shot him a look. He responded by shooting me a look and saying, "Dana" in a terse voice. Not to be outdone, I said in my best terse voice, "Doug." Yes, never let it be said that we are not two very articulate individuals! We immediately recognized the fact that the stress and exhaustion of this experience are starting to overwhelm us, and we apologized to one another. I'm just starting to feel like my body and my psyche are just about ready to raise the white flag. I find myself walking by the surgical waiting room, Doug's transplant prep room, and the ICU and being overwhelmed by the difficult memories of this experience. I then wonder what in the world I'm doing because things are going so smoothly. I should feel nothing but happiness and gratitude. I'm guessing that since I'm slowly beginning to allow myself to relax, all of the emotion and fear that I have pushed aside is starting to resurface. I think that those feelings are just screaming at me for some recognition. It's as if the emotions have taken the form of Glenn Close's character in the movie Fatal Attraction. "We won't be ignored, Dana. Deal with us, or we'll boil your rabbit." Okay, I don't have a rabbit, but I do have a cat. Use your imaginations, please. I have babbled a bit too much tonight. Don't worry about me; this is nothing that a month of binge drinking can't cure!

4/17/03

Today was another very good day. I felt better psychologically, and Doug continues to progress physically. I had an opportunity to talk to my brother last night, and I was able to clear some of my thoughts and emotions. In addition, we had a great time making completely immature and disgusting jokes—it was a great stress reliever. As far as Doug is concerned, he is now working out daily on the treadmill and the exercise bike without oxygen. It's amazing to see him work out and maintain an oxygen saturation level around 95 percent. His breathing test numbers continue to climb, and they removed half of the staples in his chest. I offered to do it with the staple remover that's in my school bag, but he didn't think it would be wise. The best news of the day is that the doctor is giving Doug a pass to go out into the world for a few hours this Saturday and Sunday. Naturally, Doug wants to go to a bookstore, and he also suggested going to see a movie. I honestly do not care what we do. In fact, I would be thrilled to just go to Walgreen's and wander aimlessly up and down the feminine hygiene aisle. That's just how desperate I am to have some time away from the hospital with him. The doctors have also given him a release date of next Tuesday. We will have to then spend another week or two in Madison, and if all goes well, we will finally be able to go home. "There's no place like home. There's no place like home." Come here Toto, Dorothy is about to strap on and those ruby slippers and GO HOME.

4/18/03

Well, you all know the line. Say it with me and share my joy. Come on, you know the line: "Doug had another good day." My emails are starting to remind me of Barry Manilow's songs: they all sound the same, but they are so strangely pleasant. Anyway, let's talk about what's his name's day. His breathing test numbers continue to climb, he continues to grow stronger, and he had the remaining staples in his chest removed. Also, during his daily chest x-ray, he was able to sneak a peek at the film. He later told me, "You wouldn't believe the x-ray. It's like I have a totally new pair of lungs." Oops, maybe we should have spent more time on the whole lung transplant concept.

4/18/03

Doug wrote this at the hospital today and asked me to forward it to everyone. Hi Everybody! Yes, it's Doug this time! I have returned from my four day tour of Dante's Inferno and rejoined the land of the sane. I first wanted to thank everybody for all of the great cards we have received over the past three weeks. Sometimes I just sit and look at them and read them over and over. I am feeling pretty good, and surprisingly, I am in little pain. Everyday I am able to walk better and use more of my muscles. Some days are very slow, and some are fast, but on the whole, since I am doing so well, my days are filled. Again, I mainly wanted to say hello myself and thank everybody who has shown such great support to me and especially to Dana. I have so many cards now, and I'm looking forward to getting home and putting together a memory box filled with everything that everyone has sent us. I will be posting more information on what this incredible experience was like for me along with a list of 1001 things I wish I had known before transplant. Thank you again so much.

Doug and the "Twins," — my friend Lynn thought up that name for my new lungs, and I like it!

4/19/03

Well, the big day on the town became the big day in the hospital. As you may or may not remember, Doug was placed on an ECMO machine shortly after his transplant. If you don't remember, it is a machine that connects two garden hoses (doctors have a different term for them) to the femoral artery, and the machine then oxygenates the blood in an attempt to rest and heal ailing lungs. After the machine is turned off, they place a drain in the leg. That drain was removed yesterday, but the site continues to drain lymphatic fluid. Today the doctor told him that if it didn't stop draining by Monday, they would have to surgically stop it. Whoa, did he just say surgery? Yes, unfortunately he did. They will sedate him and reinsert the breathing tube for a ten minute operation. The doctor explained that the breathing tube will come out immediately after the surgery, but needless to say, we were not thrilled by this news. The doctor says that it's no big deal, but Doug is scared that this "minor" thing could lead to bigger things. He's also very upset that he may be put under again. He's enjoying being healthy and sane again, and he doesn't want a tiny oozing hole to cause a bigger medical issue or a return to Dante's Inferno. So in an attempt to slow the draining, we decided to have a sedate day today (the more active he is the more active the draining is). Also, after a short while, he looks like he wet himself—a perfect way to become a social pariah in public. Anyway, we are still planning on going out tomorrow. I hesitate to tell you this because you are going to think that we are huge losers, but we are going to go to a Laundromat to do our laundry. There is a place close to the hospital that is a cyber Laundromat. I can get a chore done, and he gets an opportunity to get out without being too active. Besides, if it looks like he wet his pants, people will just think that he came to wash them. This will be our first Easter in a Laundromat, and I think this just may have the potential of becoming a tradition. I want to wish everyone a joyous and happy Easter or Passover. This is a wonderful time to celebrate life, and we will celebrate our new lives and the many blessings that God has bestowed upon us in a Laundromat. I was thinking of buying some liquid "Cheer" detergent and some plastic wine glasses for tomorrow. We can then toast one another over the washing machine and pour in our cups of "Cheer." Now that's living!

4/20/03

Well, we did indeed spend a part of our Easter Sunday in a Laundromat. But instead of sitting and waiting for the laundry, we got crazy and went to Walgreen's. No, we did not wander around the feminine hygiene aisle. We then went back to throw the clothes in the dryer and then proceeded to Barnes & Noble. Doug enjoyed the day out tremendously, and I was able to join a local gang. It seems that the only other people who were doing their laundry were a little rough. As we pulled into the Laundromat, I asked what losers (besides us) would do their laundry on Easter Sunday. Well, it seems that Madison's finest gang bangers do! Beyond our pleasant outing, the day was actually a very challenging one emotionally for Doug. He is really scared about the operation tomorrow, and the emotional magnitude of this experience is really hitting him. We spent a great deal of time talking, and I think that it helped us both. He is feeling guilty about putting me through this experience. I told him that he need not worry nor feel guilty about anything because I have always known that this would one day be my reality. I chose this path; he did not. He told me for the first time today that on the day we were married, he prayed to God to just grant me five years with him. Well, good grief, where are the tissues? I told him that God has granted us almost eight years, and it looks like he is going to grant us several more. I also told him that while he needs to deal with all of these emotional issues, he also needs to simultaneously retain his focus on just how lucky and blessed he has been. I told him that he had better get a saddle for his behind because I'm going to ride his ass about staying focused on the positive. For anyone headed down Transplant Boulevard, I must warn you that the emotional hurdles and traumas are much more intense than the physical. Doug told me today that before his transplant, he was so focused on the physical that he neglected to think about the emotional strength that would be necessary. I don't really think I fully understood just how intense this experience would be either. But I do believe that all of the experiences in our lives are lessons to be learned, and I have learned a tremendous amount about myself, my family, my husband, and my relationship with God during the past three weeks. So even though this has been the most challenging experience of my life, I thank God for it because I have grown in ways that I would have never thought possible. There has been a tremendous amount of beauty in this ugly and difficult experience, and I will forever savor the sweetness of it. Please say a prayer and keep Doug in your thoughts as he undergoes surgery again tomorrow.

4/21/03

Today was a bit of a roller coaster. Doug came through the surgery just fine, and they seem to have repaired the lymphatic leak. On the down side, the area in which they connected his new lungs to his old parts has become worse. They believe that he has some Aspergillus (a type of fungus) at this site. They feel that they can treat this, but it is a potentially serious issue. So I have no humor, insights, or philosophical ramblings for you this evening. I sit here tonight as a scared and tired woman who isn't sure if she's strong enough for this anymore.

4/22/03

It seems that my evil twin got on the computer last night. I've tried to warn her about sending emails when she's in a mood, running with scissors in the house, swimming too soon after eating, and downloading porn. All right, enough sarcasm, let's get to the point. Doug and I had a much better day today. Yesterday's news has settled, and we had an opportunity to speak with a number of doctors about the situation. Thankfully, the pack of wolves all agreed on the treatment and prognosis. Unfortunately, Dante was not on call today—seems he's doing some research in the Inferno again. Anyway, they have caught the Aspergillus at a very early stage, and they are completely confident that they can resolve the problem. The Aspergillus is currently on the surface of the tissue, and it has yet to become invasive. Perhaps the government of this country could learn something from Doug's Aspergillus. Oops, I'll stay away from politics and stay focused on the fungus. I would also like to thank everyone for all of the concern and kindness today. I received several phone calls and over sixty emails. I cannot express in words just how overwhelmed Doug and I are by the support that so many people have shown us. I feel like Sally Field on Oscar night, "You like me, you really like me." God bless you, my people. I like you too.

4/23/03

Oh, the hills are indeed alive with the sound of music, and my hotel room is alive with the sound of Doug music. Yes indeed, Doug was given an overnight pass, and he is "home" with me in the hotel. He has to go back tomorrow so that his transplant surgeon, who has been out of town, can take a final look at Doug before discharging him to the hotel. Oh, sweet freedom! After leaving the hospital today, we went to Target to pick up some junk, and then we got carry out from a pasta place. Oh, sweet nectar of life! To be able to go to a retail store and participate in good old fashioned consumerism and follow that up with a good American meal rich in carbs. People, does it get any better than this? Oh, how sweet the mundane and trivial seems after this experience. I shall not spend a great deal of time with you this evening, as I have a date. So, I bid you a very sweet adieu, and I will update you on his health tomorrow. As Doug told me this evening, "We are not discussing any part of my health tonight because this is our escape." Very well, your wish is my command, oh healthy and pink boy!

4/24/03

Are you ready to ride the roller coaster again? Today was an absolutely horrid day, and I am emotionally spent. Doug's transplant coordinator came to see us this afternoon, and her opening line was, "The results of your CT scan are not good. There is evidence of infection, there is a small area of bronchieactasis, and there may be an air leak." She followed this chipper bundle of crap news by saying, "The doctor isn't worried, and we are going to release you today." Good God woman, my brain must have an air leak because you are going to release him?????? Doug and I were speechless. We were just told yesterday that Doug's condition was excellent, and the bump in the road called Aspergillus should be managed with relative ease. What went wrong? The doctor came in shortly after she left to announce that we were free to go. Whoa, back up that trolley that just smashed our hearts, Mr. Doctor Man. We asked him to explain the CT results, and he calmly told us that the results were what they had expected to see given the Aspergillus. He told us that the patches of infection were very small and very common in post transplant CF patients. He also told us that there is definitely not an air leak. He explained that someone in CT examines the film and makes a judgment, and then the film is passed on to the doctors. He told Doug that they have seen his lungs via the bronch, and there is definitely NO AIR LEAK. As far as the bronchieactasis is concerned, it is in a small area, and they are uncertain as to why it's there. He said they will monitor it and treat it with inhaled antibiotics. They will do a bronch on him again on Monday to check everything, and they will clean out the small patches of infection. We will hopefully know more about this mess on Monday or Tuesday. In the meantime, we are free from the hospital until Monday. Please continue to keep us in your prayers because we are both feeling overwhelmed and emotionally exhausted.

4/25/03

The good news for the day is that there is no bad news today! The beauty of being released from the hospital is that no one will come knocking on your door with a big silver platter of doom and gloom. Doug and I are thrilled to be away from the house of horrors, and we are doing are best to not think about anything connected to the past four weeks—not very easy for two people who are prone to obsessing! Anyway, we had a very enjoyable day yesterday. We went shopping and ate some great Mexican food. There is nothing like a plate of Mexican food to soothe the savage beast that sometimes rages in this old Spanish teacher. On a more humorous note, I have a story to tell that will probably mortify Doug, but I'm going to tell it anyway. As you may remember, he had surgery on his leg on Monday to seal a lymphatic leak. Since that time, the surgical site has continued to ooze. Don't worry, the doctors have said that this is completely normal as long as it stays clear and shows signs of slowing each day. So let's get back to the funny part. Doug has been putting gauze and tape over the wound for several days, and while it works, it is an annoying solution because the gauze just holds the moisture in place and leaves the wound constantly moist. Well, Doug didn't just marry me for my tremendous beauty; there is also a well developed brain between these ears! I suggested that he use one of those paper thin maxi pads because it would absorb any oozing and pull the moisture away from his body. And to think he used to make fun of and be repulsed by the commercials that would show the super absorbency of the maxi pad. Well, after some serious cajoling, he consented to the idea of strapping that big old pink maxi pad to his leg. I folded it over so that it stuck on itself and then tied it on his leg with a Montgomery strip (a medical thing that is taped to the leg and has strings attached to it). Well, it worked like a charm! When we went out, he was a little nervous about it falling out, but that little sucker clung to his leg like mountain goat. So the next time you have a problem that doesn't seem to have a solution, don't overlook the power of the maxi pad.

4/26/03

I'm sitting in bed in a hotel room, and I'm wondering what I'll write to you today. There is not much to report concerning Doug's health. He feels better and stronger each day, and his breathing test numbers continue to improve. So again, what should we talk about today? How about them Cubs? No, sports talk is boring. Is anyone having any issues with regularity? No, that's disgusting and much too personal. Let's talk about life and what it means to be given a second chance. Yes, Dana, let's! For anyone who is rolling their eyes at the mere thought of a philosophical rambling, MOVE AWAY from the delete button. That's it, nice and slow, and no one gets hurt. All right, now let's chat. Doug and I had a really nice long talk last night about this whole experience, and as I related to you before, Doug is adamant that the physical challenges are nothing in comparison to the emotional challenges. First, how can you ever truly express your gratitude to the donor family? There is a pair of new lungs that have taken up residence in my husband's body, and for the first time in years, they have given him the ability to breathe and be active without restriction. These lungs shall forever be connected to a currently nameless and faceless person who once lived, loved, laughed, and cried. Who was this person? Each day, I ache for this unknown family's loss, and yet I rejoice in our good fortune. This whole process reflects the sweet and sour of life; the circle of life. One person is taken from this world, and another is given a second chance. I am also reminded of this circle of life by my own experience in the waiting room of the ICU. During the time that Doug was in the ICU, I spent countless hours in that waiting room, and over time, I got to know two other families who were sharing the lung transplant experience. Each day, we would share updates, fears, joys, and laughter. We shared a bond and an experience that few people will ever understand. As time progressed, and our loved ones improved and we were able to spend more time in the hospital rooms, we saw less of each other. But each day, as I would pass by the waiting room, it was filled with a new cast of characters, and I would see the same fearful face that I once called my own. At one point, there was a family who was waiting for their father to pass away. He had been taken off of life support, and they were waiting for his body to let go. I watched their pain for several days, and I silently felt guilty that I felt so happy for my own good fortune. I pictured Doug's donor family sitting in a hospital experiencing the same anguish, and I marveled at the amazing synchronicity of joy and sadness. I am reminded of my favorite literary passage from the book The Hours: "We live our lives, do whatever we do, and then we sleep—it's as simple and ordinary as that. A few jump out of windows or take pills; or die by accident; and most of us, the vast majority, are slowly devoured by some disease, or, if we're fortunate, by time itself. There's just this for consolation: an hour here or there when our lives seem, against all odds and expectations, to burst open and give us everything we've ever imagined, though everyone knows that these hours will inevitably be followed by others, far darker and more difficult. Still, we cherish the city, the morning; we hope, more than anything, for more." And so it is the same with the transplant experience. The journey is a dark and difficult one, but it gives us everything we've ever imagined and fills us with the promise of more.

4/27/03

I've gotten so many great responses to my updates that I thought I would treat you to a second helping today. Actually, the truth be told, I'm just plain bored silly in this Godforsaken, polyester clad, simulated wood grain hotel, and I need something to do. Doug and I did some laundry and walked around State Street in downtown Madison today. For those of you who are unfamiliar with Madison, State Street is a Bohemian collection of small shops—most of which need a good scrubbing and delousing. It's really a great place to watch people and get an infectious disease at the same time. It was an absolutely glorious day, so we also strolled along a street filled with fraternity and sorority houses, and it was then and there that I decided that I think I just may be feeling the signs of middle age. There were a tremendous number of hard bodied youngsters gracing the front porches, and I realized that my thirty-five year old boobs didn't feel or look quite as perky as they once did. While I was analyzing the evil effects of gravity, I suddenly realized that my ears were being assaulted by tremendously loud, hip hopping, bass pumping, funky music. I was mortified when I said to Doug, "Those damn kids should turn that music down." Am I ninety years old; what's wrong with me? I quickly regained my senses and realized that those young, perky, hard bodied kids were doing just exactly what Doug and I were doing: enjoying life. I don't mean to belabor the point here, but who couldn't enjoy life with bodies like that—honestly! In closing, I would like to remind everyone that Doug has his bronch tomorrow at 11:00 a.m. We are a little nervous, but I truly have a positive feeling about everything; God help me if my psychic powers are on the fritz. I would seriously appreciate your thoughts and prayers. Your support, prayers, and kind words have sustained us for the past four weeks, and I know that they will sustain us tomorrow. I look forward to bringing you very good news.

4/28/03

I am very happy to announce that I do indeed have very good news today. Doug's bronch showed signs of improvement, and the doctor even said that he did not expect to see so much improvement and that he is progressing better than others who have had the same problem. They cleaned out the area, and we were even able to see pictures of the before and after shots of the cleaning. I think it looks disgusting before and after, but the post cleaning shot does look much better. They will do another bronch on Friday to make sure that things are continuing to progress as expected. Doug also overheard the doctor say that they did a biopsy last week when they went back to check on the then suspected Aspergillus. Again, there was zero rejection. Thank you for letting us know that the CT scan looked bad and forgetting to mention that there was a biopsy. We didn't even know that they had done a biopsy last week. Grrrrrrr. Anyway, the news was very good today, and we are feeling very relieved and blessed. So despite the fact that I no longer have the boobs of a twenty year old, and my husband is still wearing maxi pads, life is very good today. Thank you again for your thoughts and prayers. God bless.

4/29/03

These updates are getting harder to do because there is currently so little to report. Doug and I took a nap, I got a hair cut, Doug threw up, I had a slight case of road rage when someone was driving too slowly for my liking, the hotel bathtub is draining a little slowly, and we feel very strongly that Clay, the contestant from the TV show American Idol, should be banished to some distant and heinous forest in Germany. That, my friends, was our day in a nutshell. Medically, I have nothing to report to you. Doug went to the hospital for two routine post transplant infusions. Want to experience gut-wrenching, mind-numbing, hallucination-provoking boredom? If so, I highly recommend three hours in the infusion "suite" at your local hospital. We did speak with Doug's coordinator today, and we talked about the "surprise" biopsy that we learned about yesterday, and it seems that she knows nothing about it either. Doug's doctor is either delusional, we are potentially delusional, or the right hand doesn't know what the left hand is doing. Either way, these people are making me crazy. Actually, it may be too late—they may have already driven me mad. Lately, I have been plagued by this overwhelming desire to purchase a white jumpsuit with arms that tie in the back so that I can go and live in a corner just inside the hospital entrance and spend my days drooling in the fetal position. Wow, I should wrap this up before I really start to scare you. Don't worry I really do still have a few shreds of sanity remaining. By the way, for everyone who has complimented me on my writing skills, have any of you noticed that I seem to have some odd aversion to paragraphs? It just dawned on me that I have been rambling for four weeks, and I have never broken my thoughts into paragraphs. I have shown complete and utter disdain for the mighty paragraph—paragraphs unite and demand representation! Oh dear, I think I have gone mad. One more thing: I shall not burden you with my craziness again until there is actually something to report. Hey, did I just hear a rousing chorus of "Thank God?"

4/30/03

I cannot believe the number of emails that I received today asking me to continue to ramble. What is wrong with you people? I am actually quite flattered that you haven't grown to find me tedious or annoying, so now the pressure is really on to entertain you. Gee, I have such performance anxiety now. Is this what it's like to be a man? I actually do have some things to report to you today. Last night, Doug noticed what looked like a blister between two staples in the incision in his leg. We spent some time analyzing it, staring at it, touching it, and discussing it. Amazingly enough, after all of that time and effort, we came to the same conclusion: we aren't doctors, and we don't know what the hell this is. So Doug called the hospital and described the mysterious creature, and the powers that be at the center of the universe (UW Madison) decided that it could wait until the morning. So this morning a nurse looked at it and said, "Hmmm, I don't think it's an infection…let me get someone else." Second nurse enters and declares, "Hmmm, I'm not really sure…I think I'll find a doctor." Do you realize just how much sarcasm I could unleash here? I'm showing so much restraint you cannot believe it. Let's get back to the story. Two residents enter the room and say, “Hmmm, it doesn’t look infected, but we’re going to page your doctor to see what he wants to do with this.” They decided that they would aspirate the mystery creature, culture it, and remove the staples. Thankfully, there was nothing to aspirate, so it seems that the creature will forever remain mysterious. Meanwhile, while examining the mystery creature, the doctors noticed the edema in his leg that has been there for two weeks. Now mind you, Doug has mentioned the swelling to anyone willing to listen ever since it appeared. Today the doctors said, “Boy, you sure have some swelling in your leg; you should really be wearing a surgical sock.” I can honestly say that I have never had a desire to tie a surgical sock around someone’s neck until today. When we asked if they could give us one, the response was, “We can’t give you a surgical sock because you are no longer an inpatient, but we can give you two ace bandages.” Is it me, or am I living in the Twilight Zone? Now, let’s fast forward to this afternoon. About 3:00, we get a call from Doug’s transplant coordinator, and it seems that his Cyclosporine level is extremely low (88 when it should be 225). His levels have been steadily dropping since they stopped a drug called Ketoconazole and replaced it with Voriconazole for the Aspergillus. It seems that Ketoconazole increases the level of Cyclosporine in the blood, so his levels have been dropping for about a week. They raised his dosage yesterday, but about an hour after he took his morning dose, he threw up. So it is highly likely that he got a very small morning dose yesterday morning and that would explain his extremely low levels today. When Doug spoke to his coordinator, he asked if he was in jeopardy of rejection, and her response was, “Yes, that’s why I freaked out when I saw your numbers.” Okay, I have held back throughout this email, but I shall now unleash. For the love of God woman, you freaked out? What are we supposed to do? Have a double freak out—maybe even a triple freak out? Run down the hotel hall screaming, “Rejection, rejection?” Go ahead and buy those white jumpsuits and let the drooling begin? Ahhhhhhhhhh. To make this already long story short, they have kept his Cyclosporine dosage the same and resumed the Ketoconazole. He will have a blood test again on Friday, and we are going to request a biopsy during his bronch on that same day—no more surprise biopsies, thank you. Oh, dear Lord, grant me the patience that has packed its luggage and abandoned me.

p.s. Screw the paragraphs.

5/01/03

I have often been accused of thinking too much. Ironically, this is a charge that I have never given much thought to until this experience. Well, today I decided that this accusation just may be legitimate. This experience has given me an incredible amount of time for thought, reflection, and introspection. From the ICU waiting room, to my husband's bedside, to the hotel room, I have been able to literally dissect every aspect of my world, and I have come to some conclusions. First, life is absolutely incredible. I have already spoken about the amazing synchronicity of life, but I continue to be astonished by it. I find myself looking at everything in a different manner. The colors now seem more vibrant and vivid; the air sweeter. It has been incredible to watch the grass turn green and the flowers bloom as nature is reborn along with my husband. But yet, I somehow feel so distant from the world. I watch people moving through their lives here, but it seems as if I am removed—a casual observer on the sidelines. I sometimes forget that Doug and I had a life before all of this. Our former world and routines now seem so distant and foreign. I honestly sometimes forget that I have a job; that we have a cat; that we have a home and a comfortable life in a town not too far from here. Doug and I were just discussing tonight that while the prospect of going home is so exciting, it is also very scary. The idea of going home and just picking up where we left off is absolutely incomprehensible to both of us. We are both such different people now, and our lives will be so different. For years, I have never felt like an adult despite the fact that I'm thirty-five years old, I have been married for almost eight years, and I have been educating teenagers for the past thirteen years. Before this experience, I had always felt like I was only playing the role of an adult. But when I looked in the mirror today, and I saw a few gray hairs and the lines that have taken up residence under my eyes during the past four weeks, I realized that I finally feel grown up, and it feels really good. Doug gets to breathe, and I finally get to feel grown up. Secondly, doctors and nurses are amazing. I have been fairly critical of some of the things that have occurred here in Madison, and I will continue to stand by this criticism. However, I am truly amazed at the intelligence, skill, and dedication of these people, and I thank God for their talents. I also thank God for every doctor who cared for Doug before his transplant, especially his doctor in Milwaukee. Doug's health was starting to deteriorate when he began to see her, and she pushed him to get listed and pushed him to take this opportunity. Her common sense, straightforward, and caring approach was just what he needed, and we can't imagine having gone through the transplant waiting period without her and the clinic nurse. Thirdly, God is amazing. What else needs to be said about that? Fourth, my family, friends, and the people of the online support groups of Cystic-L and Secondwind are amazing. I can't imagine what this experience would have been without their support. I have so many people to thank: my two good friends who sat with me during Doug's surgery while our families traveled to Wisconsin, my brother and father who kept me sane through laughter, my mom who sat and cried with me on the phone during Doug's surgery, Doug's sister and father who provided whatever I needed whenever I needed, my best friend from grade school who came to stay with me, my coworkers who took on extra work and disrupted their lives to provide a smooth transition for my classes, my students who have weathered the changes and shown me such kindness, friends who have shown such support and friendship, and everyone on the online support groups who have been supremely superb to both of us. And finally, on a much lighter side, I have learned that peanut butter in a squeeze tube and Jell-O in pre-made cups are amazing. Try living in a hotel for a while, and you'll understand what I mean.

5/02/03

Hi, everyone! Yes, this is Doug this time! I wanted to send out another thank you to everybody who sent me a card for my recent transplant. Half of all the cards I got were from people on both Secondwind and Cystic-L. It was so touching to receive cards from the people on these two lists. I cried several times just sitting and reading the cards sent from such wonderful people. I really can't tell you how much energy and hope this gave me. As anyone who has gone through this experience already knows, transplant is extremely difficult, even when things go well. I know that many other people have had more difficulties than I have had, and I can't image how deep the struggle is for them. I had to struggle on many days, and I have had a fairly good recovery. It is the hardest thing I have ever had to do, which is why the cards had such an impact on me. I felt as if with each card I was getting more and more strength. It was like the more people encouraged me, the more confident I felt in myself. So thank you, thank you, and thank you again. I will never forget how wonderfully I was treated by so many people on these two lists, and you all gave me the strength to face each day with hope and perseverance. I thank you all from the bottom of my soul.

5/02/03

The news is very, very good today. Doug had his bronch, and the Aspergillus site continues to show slight improvement. Now read this next line slowly and carefully because it's oh so fine. They are allowing us to go home. You know, "Home, home on the range, where the deer and the antelope play, where seldom is heard a discouraging word, and the skies are not cloudy all day." I've always liked that song, and it somehow seemed so appropriate to sing it on this lovely evening. It's really a shame that you are unable to see my corresponding interpretive dance. Anyway, we are planning on leaving tomorrow morning. By the time we were given the emancipation proclamation, it was late in the afternoon, and I didn't have the energy to pack up, load the car, and drive my moderately sedated husband home. We are finally ready and eager to go home and begin again. I have enjoyed sharing my thoughts and experiences with you over the course of the past month, and there is a bittersweet feeling as I write these concluding words tonight. You have allowed me to share the most profound time of my life, and in return, you have offered me nothing but love, kindness, and support. In the words of Carol Burnett, "I'm so glad we had this time together, just to have a laugh or sing a song, seems we just get started and before you know it, comes the time we have to say, so long." We have had some laughs, and I did sing a song for you this evening, so it now indeed seems appropriate to say, "So long, my friends. Doug and I have some living to do." God bless all of you—we'll be in touch.

5/27/03

Yes, just when you thought it was safe to check your email, the dreaded updates have returned to pollute your mailboxes. Doug went to Madison last Friday to have a bronch, and the results were a little disappointing. The Aspergillus site has not worsened, but it appears to be stagnating in terms of healing. The doctor removed a lot of dead tissue, but he was unable to remove all of it. So Doug is going to have debridement surgery this Friday at the anastomotic sites. Translation: Doug is going to have all of the dead crap removed from the area where his donor lung connects to his old bronchial tube. The surgery is being done on an outpatient basis, but depending on what the surgeon sees, Doug may be hospitalized this weekend for an IV anti-fungal. The doctors mentioned IV Amphotericin, but we would like to avoid that particular medication because it can be very toxic to the kidneys. I have been doing some research, and it seems that there has been a great deal of success with IV Voriconazole. So we are going to do some serious chatting with the powers that be if IV's are recommended. I'm sure that the doctors will be thrilled to have two non-doctors question their choice. Doug and I are probably every doctor's worst nightmare. We bring new meaning to the concept of being proactive in one's healthcare. Please keep Doug in your thoughts and prayers this Friday, and I will keep you updated, whether you like it or not!

5/30/03

Today's trip to Madison was a test of supreme patience. We arrived at 10:00 for his 12:00 surgery, and we were quickly whisked back to a room. Wow, such quick service, I naively thought—stupid woman. Doug's surgery was pushed back two hours because the surgeon was delayed by his morning heart surgery. They finally came to take him down at 2:00, and by 3:30, I was basking in the glow of Doug's transplant surgeon. He told me that the left anastomosis was looking better and was showing signs of healing, but there was also evidence of bronchomalacia (a weakening of the cartilage) that may require a stent. He was able to clean out the area, and they will wait for the cultures to see what freaky ass creatures will grow (those are my words, not the doctor's). They will also do a bronch in about a week and a half to check the site again, and they will then decide what course to take. For now, Doug will continue on the oral Voriconazole, and everything stays status quo. I did express my concern about the possible future use of IV Amphotericin, and the doctor mentioned a drug called Caspofungin. Damn, I couldn't match wits with the man on that drug! All of my research was on IV Voriconazole, so now I've got some new researching to do. I should just give up this Spanish teaching gig, go to medical school, and save myself a lot of grief. So the day was fairly decent, and the anesthesiologist even told us that we were a "really neat" couple. Awww, now how cute is that? Thanks for the thoughts and prayers, and we'll keep you updated.

5/31/03

I wanted to write a short note to thank everyone who responded to my last update, and I also wanted to assure everyone that I am just fine. My brother noticed that my last email contained a number of grammatical/spelling errors, so he was just convinced that these errors were a sign of something more sinister! So for anyone who was also concerned that my mistakes were a sign of a breakdown, I assure you that it was nothing more than a tired girl who is growing tired of the evil Aspergillus and the weekly trips to UW Madison. Tired girls just shouldn't be trusted to write prose. Once upon a time I said, "Screw the paragraphs," so today I shall make a new proclamation: "Screw grammar and spelling!" Take care, everyone.

6/9/03

Unfortunately, this email did not come along to brighten your mailbox's day. Doug and I are savoring the bowels of UW hospital again. Doug was doing very well after his debridement surgery, and his lung function was just skyrocketing. But on Friday, his pulmonary function tests began to dip, and he developed quite a raspy rumble in the center of his chest. When we called the hospital on Saturday, they just dismissed it as post surgery inflammation. When we called again on Sunday, they told us to wait until Monday so they could consult the physicians. Then on Monday, they called to tell us that the blood level test for Doug's anti-fungal drug had come back, and it was about 80 percent below therapeutic level. Consequently, they decided to admit him to the hospital to start an IV anti-fungal. Now, this is where Dana blows a gasket. Doug had been taking his anti-fungal drug for over a month before they drew a blood level. Since I didn't even know that they could do a blood level on an oral anti-fungal, I never questioned why they weren't checking it. The bottom line is that his level has more than likely not been therapeutic for a good month. Gee, could this be the reason that his healing was slow and eventually stagnated? I am not prone to swearing, but I have used the "F" word like a possessed trucker today. I have used it as a noun, an adjective, an adverb, and a verb. I just can't seem to say it enough. We were only able to see residents this afternoon, so my line of interrogation for Doug's doctors will have to wait until tomorrow. He will be undergoing a bronch tomorrow, and we will hopefully know more about his condition tomorrow. Please keep him in your prayers, and please say one for me because I am so angry that I'm afraid I'm going to have an aneurysm.

6/10/03

My swearing has slowed down a bit today, but my anger is still in high gear. Doug had his bronch today, and the doctor said that the anastomotic site did look better, and he believes that we are on the "right track." Well, yes, thank goodness we have finally found the right track because that was one tough track to find. Hey, anyone got a map? We're looking for the Aspergillus right track, and we just can't seem to find it. Paging Dr. Aspergillus Right Track. Anyway, the doctor also discovered some "junk," and he believes that Doug has a mild Pseudomonal infection. Paging Dr. Pseudomonas Right Track. Hey, can anyone find the right track? Damn, is right track even in the dictionary? Maybe I'm not spelling it correctly. Maybe we should do a blood test. Surely we can find the right track through a blood test. Okay, okay, I'll stop the sarcasm train. Hey, did someone mention trains? Don't trains run on tracks? But do trains run on the right track? That's really the question. Anyway, in addition to the IV anti-fungal, he has also been placed on two IV antibiotics. I did get a chance to speak to the doctor after the bronch, and I questioned him about the Voriconazole blood test issue. The conversation went a little something like this:

Doctor: "The healing does look better, and the IV anti-fungal should really speed up the healing process."

Dana: "Speaking of anti-fungals, is there any particular reason that you waited over a month to do a blood level test?"

Doctor: "Oh, I don't believe that it was a month."

Dana: "Oh, I do believe it was. I counted the exact number of days yesterday."

Doctor: "Well, it's a new drug, and well, what can I say? We didn't know any better. You know, Voriconazole is a drug that has a great deal of metabolic variability."

Dana's silent thoughts: "Oh for f...k's sake. Do I look like a doctor? How the f...k would I know that? Now I know that I'm really going out on a limb here, but do you think that metabolic variability just might justify a blood level test?"

Dana (feigning stupidity): "Do you think that the slow/stagnated healing was due to the low levels of the drug?"

Doctor: "Yes. I wanted to start him on IV's, but I couldn't convince anyone else."

I won't write my final thoughts here, but please think of the most profane and inappropriate words, and you will have successfully captured my thoughts.Final verdict on this conversation: I hate UW Madison at the moment. They are trying to kill my husband, and they are trying to create business for the psychiatric ward by driving me mad. Thank you for all of your prayers and kind words. They are helping to keep me on the right track.

6/11/03

We had a very good day today, and we had a nice long talk with the coordinator about the Voriconazole blood level and other assorted hostilities. To make a really long story short, she informed us that the two doctors dealing with Doug's case did indeed disagree on the course of therapy. One doctor thought that they needed to treat the Aspergillus more aggressively, while the other doctor thought that the treatment was aggressive enough and did not want to risk damaging Doug's liver and kidneys. So the transplant surgeon won the battle, and they stayed the course with the oral Voriconazole. As far as the blood level of Voriconazole, they did not do a test because each bronch was showing slight improvement. It was when they saw a stagnation of the healing that they decided to do the blood level check and the debridement surgery. Since the debridement surgery went well and the tx surgeon was pleased with what he saw, they saw no reason to begin IV therapy. But about a week after the surgery, Doug developed an infection, and they discovered that the Voriconazole level was too low. The doctor who originally wanted to do the IV's was apparently quick to then say, "See, we waited too long, and the inflammation created the perfect breeding ground for the Pseudomonas. I told you we should have done IV's." But the bottom line is that both doctors agree wholeheartedly that the sites look much better, and they believe that they are indeed on the "right track." In addition, Doug's coordinator told him that he is doing very well, and she is amazed at just how well he is doing despite the two infections. She said his pulmonary function test numbers are incredible, and she is sure that once the infections are cleared, he is going to be a patient that has sky high numbers. She told him that it is not the norm to see his kind of numbers just a few months after transplant. So very good! I have not sworn today, and I am back to using my good words. I no longer hate Madison, and my trust in their ability was slightly restored today. The coordinator told us that it is not unusual for the patients to get very confused when the doctors are disagreeing, and she even said that she sometimes gets confused by their banter and disagreements. So Doug and I are much better today, and most of my hostility has been purged. What can I say? I'm an overprotective wife who sometimes gets a little riled by circumstances that she can't control—so please forgive my hostile ramblings. "All aboard. The healing train has left the station and is now on track."

6/12/03

We are finally home, and it feels very good. Doug is on two antibiotics for the infection (oral Ciprofloxacin and IV Cefepime) and IV Caspofungin for the Aspergillus. The routine is not that bad because the Cefepime runs in over ten minutes, and the Caspofungin takes one hour to infuse. So he is not having an affair with the IV pole. However, it is a bit ironic because this routine seems so very familiar. We knew that there would be bumps in the road, and we were told that having a transplant is like trading one disease for another. But in some ways, we feel like nothing has changed since his transplant. We virtually live at the hospital, our condo is littered with medical supplies, and Doug is constantly taking pills and nebulizing something. Granted he can breathe like a champ, but I'm really beginning to feel sorry for the guy. In the past few months, he has had three surgeries and six bronchs. Will this joy ever end? I know that someday soon his infections will clear, and he will be able to start living his life again. But in the meantime, it is frustrating to have these new lungs and not be able to really use them to enjoy life. It's like having a new sports car in garage, but being unable to take it out on a spin to really let it show its power. This experience requires a tremendous amount of patience, but I feel like a three year old who wants what she wants and wants it now. But the important thing is that Doug is feeling much better, and his breathing test numbers are beginning to climb again. He will have another bronch in two weeks, and we will go from there. I'm fairly certain that we are still on the right track, but I wish that Doug and I could ride on the train instead of running along the side of it. We're getting tired.

6/15/03

I'm a little bored tonight, so I thought that I would share the boredom with you. Doug is doing fairly well, and the IV's are not causing him any problems. However, he does still have a bit of a wheezing/raspy sound to his lungs. It's very odd because the noise will come and go, and his infrequent cough is always dry and unproductive. On the home front, we are still in the process of adjusting to our new lives, but we feel like we are on hold until there is more of a resolution to his current infections. We went to a new church today, and it was as if the message was tailored directly to us. The speaker recounted the story of his daughter who was diagnosed with a heart valve problem shortly after her birth, and while he spoke, a picture of his baby daughter was displayed on the screen behind him. She was wearing an oxygen nasal cannula, and her tiny chest wore the battle wounds of heart surgery. The speaker stated that despite the fact that the doctors had given her only a 10 percent chance of survival, they never lost hope, and they never lost their faith. They gave their grief and fear to God, and he answered their prayers because that baby girl is now twenty-two years old. Meanwhile, Doug and I are sitting in the back row with tears just streaming down our faces. The baby's scars, the oxygen tube, and the message of never giving up and placing your burden in God's hands overwhelmed us. The two of us just seem to cry at the drop of a hat anymore. We're like two pregnant woman strung out on too much Prednisone! We have been doing our best to release our fears to God today, but it has not been an easy task. Life just hurts too much right now.

6/26/03

Doug and I made our weekly pilgrimage to Mecca—I mean Madison yesterday. It's easy to confuse the two places because the journey is always difficult and full of prayer. On a positive note, Doug was officially crowned president of the "I have had too many bronchs in three months club," and as a result, I have become the first lady of too many bronchs. Although our time in office has been short, I am going to take Hillary Clinton's lead by writing a novel about our bronch experiences. I'm tentatively going to use the title *Living Bronchs*. It will be quite a bit shorter than Hillary's book, but I'm thinking of fabricating a story about Doug having an affair with a nurse in the bronch suite to help boost book sales. Oh, I'm sorry. I should never write these emails when I'm tired. I have a tendency to ramble aimlessly in an attempt to stay awake and amuse myself. So now that I have purged my vapid banter, I shall tell you the real news of the day. Doug's bronch looked much better yesterday, and the bacterial infection has cleared. The Aspergillus site finally looks fairly clean, but they are going to keep him on the oral and IV anti-fungals to be safe. At the end of the IV therapy, his transplant surgeon will then do another debridement surgery to clean out the dead tissue that is still remaining. To quote his coordinator, "After that surgery, you should be able to be on your merry way." Unfortunately, we found out today that our merry way won't be anytime soon. Yesterday they told us that they would probably do the surgery in two or three weeks, but today we were told that we will have to wait five weeks. It seems that the surgeon is going to be out of town and has a very busy schedule. Gee, no problem, we'll just sit here doing IV's for the next five flipping weeks. We don't want to wait that long because we are concerned that the dead tissue will again provide the perfect breeding ground for another infection. When we aired our concerns to Doug's coordinator, she said that the dead tissue does increase his chances for another infection because the airway is not smooth, but she also told him not to worry about it because he is doing so well now. Hmm, and we'd like to keep it that way, thank you very much. I understand that there is nothing that can be done about the scheduling issue, but I just hope to God that he doesn't end up with another problem because of the delay. They also did a biopsy yesterday, and the results came back A1, which means that there are lymphocytes present, but they are not organized or attacking tissue—hmm, a little like the American military in Iraq at the moment. A1 can indicate an infection, rejection, or a natural response to the pollution in the environment, and since Doug just had a bacterial infection, it is possible that the lymphocytes are just residual. They will not alter his treatment, and Doug's coordinator said that it is very common for people to vacillate between A1 and A0 (no lymphocytes present). She also told him today that his x-ray looked superb and that his breathing test was awesome. Strange, no one in this house is feeling awesome at this point. Doug and I have been in a bit of a funk lately, and while we are still so grateful for this second chance at life, frustration, depression, and anger are currently the main emotions of our existence. But it does seem that the train is on the right track, has turned the corner, and is about to be on its merry way—at the end of July.

7/14/03

This is Doug. I have not written anything lately, so I thought that I would give an update. I am doing fairly well right now. My breathing tests, which I measure daily, have varied a bit lately, and I have had a bronch done about every two weeks to remove the dead tissue from the connection site between the new and old lungs. I hate doing my breathing tests because some days they are good, around 3.00 FEV1, and other days they are a little low, like 2.60 FEV1. I never know what to expect. I feel fine and walk for about twenty five minutes, six days a week, but my numbers are still quite erratic. It is very annoying. But overall, I feel very lucky and grateful for what I have. I have gone through a bit of a depression lately, but I am getting better psychologically. I am finally beginning to see how fortunate I really am, and I am so glad I am that I had this transplant. It has been the hardest thing I have ever gone through; I feel as if I died and was then resurrected. It is very strange process, and even though I logically know that I am in a better spot today than I was a year ago, there are some times when I feel completely overwhelmed. A great deal of my depression is from the Prednisone, so I know that it will work itself out and eventually go away. It's amazing what I can do now, compared to three months ago, when my lung function was at 16 percent. Since my life is tied up with my health right now, the hardest thing that I have had to do is to get back into my life. This has been a tremendous struggle, and I am only now beginning to pick up the pieces and move forward. It is very difficult to avoid the temptation to become consumed by and obsessed with the medical routine. But in the past few weeks, I have stopped worrying so much about everything, and I am getting back to normal. I know that it will be a slow process, and I want it to be faster. So I hope everyone is doing well, and I will keep you updated. Again, thank you so much for all of the cards and well wishes in April and May. It was so touching to receive them, and they really lifted my spirits

7/18/03

Well, it has been a while since we have chatted, and I know that you are just itching for some Doug information. Three weeks ago Doug had a bronch and a biopsy which determined that he had A1 rejection (lymphocytes present, but no active rejection). Okay, fine. But a few weeks ago, Doug's breathing test numbers began to decline, and Madison decided to have the boy come in for another bronch and biopsy. Okay, fine and dandy. When the doctor went down into Doug's lungs, there was a lot of loose goop in the area where he had the Aspergillus, so he cleaned out the goop and decided that a biopsy wasn't necessary. Okay, very fine and very dandy. After the bronch, Doug's breathing tests immediately went back up, but after only a few days, they began to fall again. This time, Madison decided that they wanted to admit him immediately to do another bronch and biopsy. When Doug questioned why it was necessary to be admitted immediately, the response was, "You might be having a rejection episode, and we may start IV steroids tonight." Okay, I'm getting worried. So off to Madison we journeyed late yesterday afternoon. We arrived in the city of doom at 6:30, but since the computers were down, they could not officially admit him, and they sent us to a care initiation wing. Okay, this is annoying. Well, well, well, we spent four hours in the care initiation wing, and when the resident finally came to see us, she informed us that they had no intentions of doing anything until after the bronch the next day. Okay, good thing we rushed over here. At 10:30, we were finally shown to our transplant suite in the transplant wing. When we arrived, one of our favorite nursing assistants came in to greet us, and she said, "Where have you guys been? We were told that you would be here around 7:00. We eventually found out that you were stuck in the care initiation wing, but we don't know why they wouldn't send you over." Okay, I'm too tired to process the stupidity of all of this. The next morning we attempted to talk about some of our frustrations about Doug's care during the past few months, but we had little success. We began by talking to the resident, and she told us that she would relay the message to the doctors. Okay, sure you will. We then talked to the coordinator, and she told us to talk to the pulmonologist. We then talked to the pulmonologist, and he told us to talk to the surgeon. Okay, for the love of God. We surrender. They finally took Doug to have his biopsy this morning, and we were told that we would have to wait seven hours for the results. Okay, a seven hour wait sounds fun! In the meantime, we returned to Doug's room and dealt with a nurse who was new to the transplant wing. She had trouble with Doug's meds, and while she was listening to his lungs, she was scanning his back like she was looking for lost luggage. She finally looked up and said, "Where is your scar?" Without missing a beat, Doug flipped up the front of his shirt and said, "Uh, that would be on the front of my chest." The nurse giggled, took a peak, and said, "Oh, there it is!" Yep, there it is. Okay, I'm out of sarcasm. After seven hours of fun and frivolity, we were told that Doug's biopsy was A0 (no rejection). Okay, most excellent. It seems that the goop from the Aspergillus site is again compromising his airways. Okay, compromised airways don't seem like a problem. Okay, I'm not out of sarcasm. We will now wait until July 28th to have the debridement surgery to remove the goop that the pulmonologist cannot. Okay, I have finished.

7/23/03

Doug and I are once again hospitalized in Madison. As all of you know, his breathing tests have been jumping around quite a bit. After his bronch and negative biopsy last week, his breathing numbers were still going up and down. So they brought Doug in again on Tuesday to do formal testing, and his numbers have now dropped 49 percent from their baseline (they had dropped 22 percent two weeks ago). They also did a CT scan, and the results were normal. The doctor said that it still does not appear that Doug is having a rejection episode, but they don't know what is going on. As a result, they hit him with a 500 mg Prednisone IV burst last night. When we asked about the debridement surgery, we were told that we would likely still have to wait until Monday. Doug feels well, has no shortness of breath, no temperature, no cough, and is saturating between 97-99 percent. Unfortunately, Doug's surgeon and pulmonologist are currently out of town. It's frustrating because the pulmonologist stated last week that he thought that the dead tissue in the anastomotic sites was causing the problem. But at the same time, he said that Doug probably didn't need to have the debridement surgery. Huh?? Our coordinator told us that the pulmonologist's note were confusing to her as well, so I know that we are not insane. Doug and I are doing fairly well, and we are quite simply too drained and exhausted to raise our eyebrows anymore. Beam me up, Scotty.

7/23/03 part II

Doug will be getting another 500 mg burst of Prednisone today, and tomorrow they will either do a final 250 or 500 mg burst. We spoke to Doug's respiratory therapist today, and we filled her in on all of the details. She told us that it is quite possible that the sloughing material and floppy airways could cause the drop in Doug's breathing numbers. She explained that the airways can essentially collapse whenever air is pushed out. But as we all know, the flipping surgery that will give us that answer will definitely not occur until Monday. When I asked the coordinator about the floppy airways, she said that it is a possibility, but as the transplant surgeon always says, "If it looks and smells like rejection, it's rejection." Hmm, and as I always say, "If it looks and feels like a pain in my ass, it must be UW Madison."

7/23/03 part III

I'm insanely bored in the hospital, so I thought that I would treat you to a third helping of Shakespeare's tragedy in a hospital. The day can be summarized as follows:Question of the day: What is wrong with Doug?

A. Respiratory Therapist's answer: "It could be a result of floppy airways."

B. Coordinator #1: "It looks and smells like rejection. We won't know if the airways are floppy until the debridement surgery is completed. The surgeon will have to remove the dead tissue before he can make a really good assessment of the airways."

C. Coordinator #2: "There are no floppy airways. The pulmonologist said that the airways are open. I understand that you guys are confused because it's so hard to filter what everyone tells you." Yes, Doug and I do need an interpreter because we are just as dumb as a box of rocks. Heck, we could barely find our way out of the parking garage to get to the hospital.

D. Transplant Doctor: "I honestly don't know what is wrong. It doesn't look like rejection, but we don't know what is causing this. Doug does have a floppy airway, and that could be contributing to the problem. However, we wouldn't expect to see such a drop in breathing numbers due to floppy airways unless he had already had a number of rejection episodes and infections."

I honestly couldn't help wondering why two and a half months of a severe Aspergillus infection, a Psuedomonal infection, a debridement surgery and ten bronchs to clean the area wouldn't fall into that category. Thanks for letting me bend your ears three times today, and I shall bend them again tomorrow because I AM SO BORED, and Doug is not providing nearly enough entertainment for my needy mind (that's a joke). By the way, Doug is scheduled to be released tomorrow barring any disasters.

7/24/03

Doug and I are home again, and we don't know anymore about his condition than when we entered the hospital on Tuesday. The doctor just doesn't know what is causing the problem, and they will wait to see what the rigid bronch will show on Monday. The doctor did tell us that IF this is a rejection episode, it could take up to a week before Doug's breathing tests show any improvement. We are nervous about this whole situation, and we are both feeling fairly worn and frazzled. I have been sleeping on a chair for the past two evenings, so I'm a little sleep deprived, and my back feels like it has been beaten with wet rags. No, I have never been beaten with wet rags, but I would imagine that the sensation would resemble the feeling I currently have. I will update as soon as we know anything.

7/28/03

Doug's surgery is at 2:15 central time today. I would appreciate any and all prayers, meditations, incantations, thoughts, chanting, and surgery dances for him. Thanks again for all of your support, and I will send an update this evening.

7/28/03

Well, I don't even know where to begin. The day got off to a bad start when we were told that the surgery was going to start a little late. And if that bundle of chipper news was not enough, we were also told that a different surgeon would be performing the bronch. Apparently, the scheduled surgeon was caught up in a meeting, and they were uncertain as to whether he was going to be able to get away in time for Doug's surgery. Hello, caught up in a meeting? We waited five weeks to get this specific surgeon, and now he is in a meeting? We were politely told that it didn't matter because the doctor who would be performing the surgery was the master doctor's partner. As it turned out, the master surgeon did escape from his meeting in time to do the surgery. Doug was gone for almost two hours before the doctor came to see me. He told me that he was a bit shocked at the condition of Doug's right airway. It seems that the cartilage in his right bronchus had broken down, and as a result, the airway was severely weakened. Since having your airway collapse is a really bad thing (sarcasm alert), the doctors immediately placed a stent to maintain the airway. They also took a chest x-ray to make sure that his right lung was not collapsing. Apparently, when an airway collapses, the lung doesn't have a mind of its own, so it just follows the leader. Thankfully, there were no signs of a lung collapse, and the doctor is confident that the stent will resolve the airway issue. I did talk to the doctor about the fact that we were extremely angry that we had to wait five weeks for the procedure, especially since we had spent the past three weeks saying, "Ummmmm, something is wrong." He looked a bit perplexed and said, "Well, did you cancel a couple of appointments within that timeframe?" I responded calmly by saying, "No, in fact, we have been begging for this procedure for past two weeks. Remember when Doug was hospitalized twice in the past two weeks and your team performed two bronchs and treated him for rejection despite the fact that his biopsy and CT scan were negative and he had no clinical symptoms? And remember those times that we kept asking about his floppy airway and were dismissed every time we brought up the subject? We wanted the procedure then, but your team told us that it could wait. And besides, as we all know, if it looks and smells like rejection, it's rejection." The doctor's response was that there was apparently a bit of a communication problem. Since he does not do the regular bronchs, he has to rely on another doctor to convey any and all information. He assured me that that particular doctor had made no mention of the severity of Doug's problem. He continued by saying that the issue must have happened recently because the other doctor would have seen it otherwise. Oh good God, Doug lost 49 percent of his lung function during the past three weeks. I don't think that this is something that happened yesterday. Needless to say, I am crazy angry again, and we are trying to decide what action we are going to take. While Doug and I were waiting to be admitted to the hospital, I started ranting like a trucker, and one of the nurses told me on our way to Doug's room that I should really contact patient relations. I intend to do exactly that, and I believe I shall be sharing my feelings with the "team." I am planning a fire and brimstone approach—a bit of a scorched earth policy—make that a scorched transplant team policy. Doug and I have lost some of our confidence in our transplant team, and I must say that that is a scary place to be. Doug is in the middle of some serious complications, so we cannot just pickup and leave this hospital. Doug is feeling well this evening, and we should be able to go home tomorrow. Unfortunately, he has another bronch on Friday so that they can check the status of the stent. If they are not happy with the stent's performance, they will replace it with the bigger one that they special ordered today. I am feeling insanely calm this evening, and I'm beginning to wonder if this place has broken my spirit. Well, if it isn't broken, it's definitely dented. I'm so tired, and I never know if I should scream, cry, or laugh at all of this. It all seems just too absurd to be true. But it is true, and it is our reality, so we will continue to deal with all of it. Thank you so much to everyone who emailed prayers and well wishes today. It was absolutely wonderful to see over thirty emails wishing us the best this evening. Doug and I could not have endured this comedy/tragedy of errors without your support. God bless all of you.

7/29/03

Doug is feeling well today, and we are enjoying the fact that he now has functioning airways. You just have to love those bronchi. Bronchi are our friends! I have just finished my letter to the patient relations department, and I am confident that we are going to get some things resolved. I was ready to lose my temper with someone yesterday, but that is honestly just not my style. I have calmed down. Actually, I think that I am calm because my adrenal glands have been on overdrive for four months, and I'm fairly certain that they just self-combusted yesterday—poof—no more adrenal glands. Anyway, I prefer the logical, calm, sequential approach to conflict resolution. It's just a part of my good old anal retentive nature. During the past three days, I have received over one hundred emails, and there is just no way that I can respond to each one personally. So I am sending out a collective thank you. Everyone has been so kind to us, and you have truly nurtured our souls and minds. I continue to be amazed by the kindness and support that we have received during the past four months, and I hope that when my constantly sedated Doug no longer needs me as his protector and guardian, I will have the opportunity to return the kindness. Thank you again. You are all very tremendous human beings, and Doug and I are very lucky to have you in our lives.

7/30/03

Since my emails are often full of depressing drivel, I thought that I would share a little joy with you this evening. Doug and I went out to dinner tonight, and then we went to the grocery store. Stay with me, I'm getting to the good part. As we were making our way to the grocery store, it began to pour. I made a mad dash for the door, and when I turned around to see where Doug was, he was also sprinting toward the entrance. Doug and I have been together for nine years, and I have honestly never seen him run. When he got to the door, we both burst into laughter. Doug said, "Good grief, I just ran. I haven't done that in so long; I really had to concentrate on how to do it." We just stood in the rain and laughed, and it was honestly the best experience that we have had since his transplant. Welcome back to your lives, Doug and Dana.

8/1/03

This email will require no post reading antidepressants or stiff drinks to numb the news. Doug had his bronch today, and the stent is in perfect position and is functioning perfectly. Doug and I did inquire about putting in the larger stent, but the doctor told us that they were lucky to get the smaller stent into position in the first place. They may place a larger stent down the road when the airway is more stable, but for now they are more than pleased with our small stent friend. See, size does not matter. Since we have received such great news today, Doug and I are going to start driving, and we won't stop until we find rain. We're looking to do some wind sprints in the rain again.

8/10/03

My friends, it is once again time for another episode of the Doug and Dana soap opera. As you know, there have been many episodes to this saga: As the Lung Turns, Days of our Lungs, All My Lungs, General Lung Hospital, etc. Yesterday, Doug started running a low fever grade fever (99.4). We were slightly concerned, but since it did not budge up during the day, we decided to just keep an eye on it. This morning, his temperature rose to 99.6, and he then started to vomit. He got so upset about the vomiting that he started to hyperventilate. Oddly enough, I just took a course on stress management last week, and I can say with great pride that I apparently learned nothing because I was completely stressed by the situation. I did manage to get Doug to the couch, and after several attempts, I did manage to calm him down. I then decided to play triage nurse, and I took his vital signs. His oxygen saturation level was good, but his pulse was pushing 150. I believe that mine was pushing 300. I also took his temperature again, and it had soared to 100.6. Okay, time to go on a road trip to Madison. When we arrived at the emergency room, Doug's temperature was 102.9. The started him on IV fluids, gave him Ibuprofen, took blood cultures, took an x-ray, and started him on an IV antibiotic. His temperature finally began to tumble back down after a few hours, and after about four hours, his temperature fell back to normal. At this point, they have no idea what is causing this. His chest x-ray looks clear, and nothing abnormal has shown up in the other tests. Therefore, we are again residing in Chateau de Madison, and we have no idea how long we have reservations. Doug and I are tired beyond belief, and Doug even thinks that I am starting to look bad! He says that he is worried about me and that I look too tired. He says that my eyes don't look right. Quite honestly, I'm a little worried about myself too. I feel as old as Methuselah, and apparently I'm beginning to look like him as well. I would again ask that you keep us in your prayers as we fight this next battle—whatever it turns out to be. I will keep you posted.

8/11/03

We found out this morning that Doug has a bacterial infection in his bloodstream, and the doctors believe that it originated in the PICC line that he has had for several months. They are treating him with two IV antibiotics, and the good news is that he is feeling much better today. He has not had a temperature since yesterday afternoon, his pulse has dropped, and he is no longer vomiting. The doctor told us that this is treatable and that they are encouraged by the fact that he has responded so well and so quickly to the antibiotics. If anyone has a success story of a bloodstream infection, please share it with us. We could use some encouragement.

8/11/03 part II

Look out, she's in the hospital again, she's bored, and she's got a computer. I really have very little to say this evening, but I have nothing else to do, and these white hospital walls are closing in on me quickly. Doug is doing very well today, and he is getting restless—a very good sign. The doctors pulled Doug's infected PICC line today, and they will replace it tomorrow. They also did a CT scan, and the doctor called the results unremarkable. I normally wouldn't call the word unremarkable a good thing, but in this case, it's wonderful. Having your face described as unremarkable is bad, but having your CT scan described as unremarkable is profoundly good. The doctor will do a bronch on Wednesday to check his stent and clean it out if necessary. It will be a bit like having the tidy bowl man clean his lung bowl. The doctor will brush around a bit and flush out the unnecessary. We are hoping that his lungs will be sparkling fresh, and we are hoping to hear the word unremarkable again. The doctor also said that they will release him after the bronch if he continues to do well. Well, that is all for the evening edition of life in the lung prison. Until tomorrow, my remarkable friends.

8/12/03

I have absolutely nothing to relate to you this evening. Doug still feels well, and I am still bored silly and sleep deprived. The good news is that I'm so tired that I have become slaphappy. Doug and I got a little giggly last night at bedtime, and we had to shut the door to avoid disturbing the other patients. We're not sure, but we believe that is actually a federal crime to laugh in a hospital. Damn it, you are in a hospital, put on your grim face and suffer. Doug and I were thinking of performing a modified version of Christmas caroling in the hospital corridors this evening to lighten the mood of this place. We're going to go door to door and sing to anyone who will listen. We are still in the process of selecting our playlist, but we are definitely including, "Swing Low Sweet Chariot," "Nobody Knows the Trouble I've Seen," and my solo rendition of "Baby Got Back" for the male patients. We're really excited about the potential of becoming lounge singers at UW Madison. This new singing gig could lead to really big things for us! I need to end this inane little email. Doug has the bronch that was already scheduled last week tomorrow afternoon, so we would again appreciate all thoughts and prayers. After the bronch, we will meet with the coordinator and the head surgeon to discuss some "communication" issues that we have had in the past. God willing, the bronch and the meeting will go smoothly, and we will be able to take our new lounge act on the road very soon.

8/13/03

Okay, you are going to want to go to the bathroom, get a snack, or find a comfortable chair before you read today's update. I'll give you a minute. All right, everyone settled? Gather around me children, and I'm going to tell you a nice long story. The day began this morning when the transplant surgeon unexpectedly popped into our room. We were supposed to meet with him and the coordinator in the afternoon after Doug's bronch, but he was afraid that his surgical schedule would preclude the meeting. So we began the process of dissecting all of the issues that have taken place in the past four months, and to make a really long story short, he admitted that there were some significant issues of communication. He also admitted that UW is not a perfect place and that there is plenty of room for improvement. I must admit that this was a big concession. I was honestly prepared for the, "You just don't understand the big bad medical world, little missy." But he took complete and full responsibility for all of the issues and told us that things will definitely improve in the future. The surgeon also said that he is relinquishing the heart program, and he will now only be focusing on the lung program. Whooohooo, more time for us! He also told us that he and the other surgeon will be doing Doug's bronchs until the airway is more stabilized. He explained that the staff pulmonologists don't always see things in the same way that surgeons do, and given the complexity of Doug's case, the surgeons will be handling things for a bit. I could really be sarcastic and nasty here, but I shall not. I will be staying positive tonight, boys and girls. We also got a bit more detailed explanation of Doug's problem today, and it seems that his right bronchus actually has a hole in it (Doug has been singing the Hank William's song "My Bucket's Got a Hole in It" since hearing the news), and the donor tissue that is wrapped around the anastomosis has been flopping down into the hole and blocking the airway intermittently. The doctors tried to remove the flopping tissue, but they were afraid to yank too hard because it is so close to the pulmonary artery. Apparently, the transplant team had a similar case that resulted in what the doctor called, "an unfavorable outcome." Translation: they nicked the pulmonary artery, and the poor guy died. Oops. As a result, the doctors decided to leave Doug's flopping piece of tissue alone and place the stent to strengthen the weakened airway. They are planning to leave the stent in place for at least a few months, and they are fairly confident that the hole in the bronchus should heal/seal itself in time. If Doug ends up needing the stent for a longer period of time, the doctor said that they may put in a larger one to open the airway as much as possible. It seems that Doug has a fairly large airway. Wow Doug, that sure is an impressively big airway! Why, I've never seen such a big airway! I really felt good about the meeting, and I honestly believed that the issues with the transplant team had been resolved. We were also assured that things will change, and if not, the supervisor provided us with her direct number. Okay, Dana is happy, and things are finally going to start to go smoothly. Oh Dana, you are so stupid. Let's move along to part two of our story. As you know, Doug was supposed to have another bronch today at 1:00 to check the status of the stent. Doug was taken down to the surgery prep room, the nurses did their thing, and the anesthesiologist even bolted into the room to say that it was time to go to the operating room. Great, we are going to be early! Wrong, the surgery is going to be delayed two hours. Huh? The anesthesiologist's explanation was as follows: "The doctor can't do the procedure in the outpatient operating rooms. He may have to do more invasive surgery, so he needs to perform the surgery in the main operating room." Huh? The surgeon just told us that the CT scan of the stent looks beautiful. More invasive surgery? Huh? We were escorted back to Doug's room, and Doug immediately called his coordinator. Five minutes later, the doctor blew into the room and said, "You're going to like this story." Doug and I looked at one another and said in stereo, "Doubt it." To make his long story short, the doctor has to spend so many hours per week at the VA hospital next door, and Wednesdays are his day to do so. Given that information, we don't know how in the world Doug's bronch even got scheduled for that time in the first place. Insert profanity and move forward. We were then told that the bronch would take place at 3:00. Grrrrr. Insert more profanity and proceed. Now here's the funny part (sarcasm alert): Doug was not taken down for his bronch until 6:30. Isn't that hilarious? Can you hear my laughter? Yes, it's the sound of sheer insanity. You can't hear it, but I'm cackling like a hyena on crack. I swear I have lost my mind. It's gone, and I'll never get it back. Goodbye, my mind. You have served me well. Run, be free. That's it, run, run like the wind and escape from this hospital. Let's move on to part three. The doctor finally did the bronch, and the stent looked good and was in position. However, there was apparently a rather large mucous plug that occluded the majority of the stent. Doug just did his lung function tests this morning, and they had jumped back up to 70 percent. Before the stent was placed, they had dropped to 41 percent. Given the fact that the stent was so occluded, the doctor was amazed that his lung function was so high. He told me that his numbers should easily go back to his baseline now that the airway is open for business again. We are also free to go home now, but it is after 8:00, and Doug still has another good hour in the recovery room. I'm not certain if we will leave this evening, but if Doug is willing, we're going to bust a move for the doors. I have been sleeping in a chair for three days, and I am drooling over the thought of sleeping horizontally in a real honest to goodness bed. Thanks for sticking through the saga this evening—it has been a very long day.

8/14/03

Doug and I are home today after arriving around 10:00 last night. Our bed felt great, but I feel like I am in the midst of a drunken stupor this morning. I have honestly never been drunk in my life, but I would imagine that this is what it feels like. See, this is why I don't drink—it hurts. Thankfully, there is no new news to share in regard to Doug's health, but I do have a little rambling that I feel compelled to share with all of you. I have been sending these emails to family, friends, and our online support groups during the past four months, but this note is specifically for the individuals from our support groups. However, I am also sending it to our family and friends because I want everyone to hear what I have to say. Silence, everyone. When we were speaking to the surgeon during our "conference" yesterday, he made a few statements that I thoroughly enjoyed, and I wanted to share them with you. He began by telling us that the decision to have a lung transplant is a very tough one because it is a very long, arduous, and uncertain journey. He described the individuals who are willing to attempt the journey as "very hardy souls." He continued by saying that he has done about 450 lung transplants, and he has always found that the individuals with CF are the toughest of the bunch. He explained that since they have been in the medical system for so many years, they know how to get what they want, and they have also developed a fairly significant distrust of the system. A distrust of the system? What is he talking about? Can someone explain what he means by this?!!!! Finally, he told us that individuals with CF tend to fair the best in lung transplantation because they know how to monitor their health, and they know how to manipulate and work the medical system. I agree with the doctor wholeheartedly, but I would like to add a few a thoughts to the mix. Since I'm speaking to an audience of people with cystic fibrosis, I would like to share my thoughts and feelings about all of you. I could not agree more with the surgeon's statement that people with CF are very hardy souls. You have been given a cruel and relentless disease, and no one will ever know (in this life) why you have to endure so many daily challenges and heartaches. But I do believe that there can be tremendous meaning and opportunities for growth and learning in the suffering, and I believe that the challenges you face can ultimately make you stronger. I must say, however, that Doug and I have reached a point in which we feel strong enough, thank you very much! We don't want to grow and learn anymore! We're good, thanks. Just leave us alone now—no more growing and learning necessary here! But seriously, I am constantly amazed and uplifted by the courage and strength that I continually see you exhibit in spite of the constant uncertainty of your lives. I am also amazed by the grace, class, and humor that shines through despite the weight of your illness. Doug is the most amazing man I have ever met, and I can say without reservation that the people I have "met" on the CF support lists are equally amazing. You are very special souls, and anyone who is fortunate enough to be in your lives is very blessed indeed. So on this lovely day, I want to publicly say that I admire all of you tremendously. I admire your courage, your tenacity, your humor, and your determination to battle this illness and live your lives. You can't see me, but I am tipping my hat to all of you. I'm wearing a Carmen Miranda fruit salad hat right now, and I would like to mention that it is no easy task tipping this kind of hat. But for you, I will do anything. I admire you, and I am so very proud of all of you. Keep fighting the good fight. And for those who support and stand beside the people with CF, stay strong and know that you are not alone. Please know that there is value in this struggle, and even though I feel tattered and beaten, I would not trade the past four months for anything. Despite the hard road, Doug and I are still here, and we are much better people as a result. Our relationship has deepened, and our hearts have softened. Life is very hard, but life is so very sweet, and we look forward to savoring whatever it may hand us for many years to come.

8/26/03

Doug had another bronch today and things went very well. Thankfully, there are not many details to share. His left anastomosis has healed, and the right one is well on its way. The doctor said that he was a bit surprised to see so much improvement in just two weeks. To quote the doctor, "I can finally say that I am confident that we are winning the war." Very good, doctor. Your words are sweet music to my tired ears. Doug and I shall finally declare a small victory.

8/30/03

Well, shit. If there is an email with Doug's name and a date, it can't be good. That's right, Doug and I are once again hospitalized in Madison. What's wrong? Oh, who the hell knows? He started running a low grade fever this morning, and it eventually went to 101.3. But just as quickly as it rose, it went back to normal. So, Doug now has no fever and is feeling fine. Until they have more answers, they have him on three antibiotics. We are frustrated beyond belief, and we cannot believe that we are here AGAIN. We are praying that this is not due to Madison's most recent mistake with one of Doug's meds. The last time he was an inpatient, they cut one of his rejection meds in half to help raise his white blood cell count. Oops, they then forgot to tell us to raise it again, so Doug was on the incorrect dose for nine days. We questioned his coordinator about the dosage the day after his release, but she had not been given the discharge orders. As a result, she told him to continue with the lower dose until further notice. Since we received no further notice, we assumed that the lower dosage was the correct dosage. Well, it seems that there was a screw up on the floor, and the coordinator never received the discharge sheets. And unfortunately, she forgot to check with the doctors about the correct dosage. It wasn't until Doug's blood test showed a high white blood cell count that the mistake was caught. But don't worry, we had another meeting with the transplant supervisor yesterday, and she apologized and gave us two $5 gift certificates. She also said that there just seems to be a dark cloud over our heads. Dark cloud, my ass! It's called the dark temple of doom that doubles as a hospital. I'll stop there because there is just too much material that I could unleash from my vault of sarcasm. I will keep you updated as we become enlightened. Sorry for the profanity, but I seem to be losing my ability to be calm and appropriate. Damn it.

8/30/03

It is one o'clock in the morning, and I can't sleep. Writing soothes me, so I thought that I might find a bit of solace and comfort in the keyboard of this computer. I have a chair that folds down into a bed this time, and despite its relative comfort, I am unable to find any peace or rest in its arms. My chair/bed is situated under a window in which I can see Doug's old ICU wing. They are in the process of remodeling the ICU and the transplant floor, so there is only the eerily golden glow of a construction lamp and the remnants of the ceiling that has been torn away. It amazes me that our lives revolved around that place only five months ago. I still have so many emotions that will be permanently connected to it. Some of the memories are sweet, and some of them are still tucked in the recesses of my mind, for they are still too painful to recount. And while all of the memories seem so fresh and new, they are also a bit faded around the edges. I'm grateful for the fact that the mind has a way of softening and fading the memories that hurt too much. And I'm glad that the place that held those difficult memories is now gone. That old ICU will be replaced by new walls, new floors, and new colors. And more importantly, new transplant patients will come and go just as we did. Soon, many other families will have their own bittersweet experiences to carry for the rest of their lives. When Doug entered that ICU five months ago, it was snowing. But as he progressed, the trees that were barren outside of his windows began to blossom, and they were soon covered in a sea of green leaves. And today, as I looked upon those same trees, they are now beginning to show the first hint of fall color. I wonder where the time has gone. We have come so far, but in some ways, it feels like we haven't moved an inch. I can't help wondering when this hospital will relinquish its hold on us. Where is our new life? This new life taunts and teases us like a playground bully. We are able to elude him for short periods of time, but just as soon as we think we have escaped his grip, the bully drags us back for another round of disappointment. Our emotions remind me of that ceiling in the ICU. They are exposed, torn, and jagged. But time renews, and I cling to that belief. The ICU will soon be new, the trees outside of the window will have new leaves this spring, and Doug and I will have that elusive promise of a new life. Thanks for letting me bend your ear with my late night ramblings. I just knew that I could share this with you.

8/31/03

After last night's rambling, I have decided that my mind is much like a television set. It needs to be turned off before I go to bed. I don't know what it is about this place, but it just makes my mind go on overdrive, and as a result, you get to read an excessive amount of drivel. We spoke to Doug's transplant surgeon this morning, and Doug has another bloodstream infection from the PICC line that is being used for his anti-fungal medication. They believe that this infection is most likely the remnants of his previous infection, and instead of immediately replacing the line, they will pull it and leave him line free for at least a week. To quote his doctor, "Your vascular tree needs a rest, and your system needs to be able to completely rid itself of the infection." It sounded much more complex and profound when he described it, but that's the gist of his conversation. They also did a CT scan last night to make sure that his stent/anastomotic site was not the issue, and the surgeon said that his lungs and the stent look perfect. He also said that although sepsis is a very serious issue, of all of the problems that this could have potentially been, this is the least serious. He also told Doug that he doesn't seem to have much luck. Hmm, I don't believe that I'll comment on that one.

9/1/03

Doug was indeed liberated today, and we are now home. He feels great, and all seems to be going well for now. End of story? Dear God, please say yes.

9/28/03

Since I have recently received a few emails asking about Doug's progress, I thought that I would take a few minutes to update everyone. Doug and I are still alive and kicking. I just looked down and noticed that my chest is still rising and falling with each breath, and the mirror that I just stuck under Doug's nose did indeed show a touch of condensation. Yes, Egor, "They're alive, they're alive." Doug is doing well, and he goes to Madison tomorrow for a bronch so that the doctor can do a biopsy and also check the status of his airways. This will be the first time in three weeks that we have made a trip to Dante's Inferno. This is the longest period of time since his transplant that we have been away from the temple of doom, and it has been absolutely wonderful. We are hoping to break our three week record very soon. Never let it be said that we are not goal oriented. Doug has returned to work, and he loves every minute of it. He has returned to his position as the social butterfly at Barnes and Noble, and all of the women seem to be elated that chatty Doug is back in the hen house. He is working only two days a week for about three hours each day. The doctors have not given him permission to do much more than that since they want him to ease back into things slowly. I returned to teaching at the end of August, and I don't seem to experience the same sense of elation that Doug does when he goes off to work. It is good to have a routine again, but getting up at the crack of dawn and entertaining the hormone bags that litter my classroom each hour is downright exhausting. My back and feet are not happy at the end of the day, but by George, the youth of Wales, Wisconsin have been educated. Well, that's about all from the chateau de lung. I will send out an update after Doug's bronch if there is anything to tell. Otherwise, I will send out a note on Tuesday after we get the biopsy results.

9/30/03

Doug had his bronch yesterday, and his biopsy showed zero rejection! He will have to have another bronch in two weeks because the doctor is thinking about removing the stent. He is either going to remove the stent completely or replace it with a bigger one. As you may or may not remember, the stent that was originally placed was too small for Doug's airway. Doug apparently got the McDonald's super size bronchus, and it needs a super sized stent. After his tiny stent was placed, his surgeon special ordered a larger stent in case the smaller stent didn't perform well. Well, the stent has performed well, but there is apparently a bit of tissue granulation just distal to the anastomosis. Dear God, I sound so smart when I use my big medical words. Too bad I have no clue what I'm talking about. Anyway, they want to monitor this granulation, and as a result, they are giving serious consideration to removing the offending stent. I'm going to ask if I can have it after they remove it. I want to create a stent earring or a stent broach—I just can't decide. I'm thinking about starting a new business venture—medical waste jewelry. Umm, actually that's a big lie. I've got to stop slamming vodka shots while writing these emails. The heavy liquor clouds my thinking. Don't worry, I'm not really drunk. I'm just drunk on the pure joy of zero rejection!

10/09/03

Doug and I received a letter today from his donor's family. I'm the one who always gets the mail, and I didn't even think twice when I began to open yet another envelope from UW Madison. But I was stunned to read the cover letter that stated that a note from the donor family was enclosed. There was a twinge of excitement, but that excitement was coupled with a nervous twinge of pain. I paused and savored the last moments of ignorance before unfolding the letter. It was written by the donor's sisters, and they generously gave us a glimpse of who their brother was and offered us more information and a photograph if we so desired. The previously unknown man who had so unselfishly returned my husband's future was now real. I thought that it would feel good to know more about him, but I can honestly say that it just hurt—profoundly. The pain and loss of their brother was clearly evident, but the two sisters wanted us to know that their brother had always been an organ donor and that he would be so happy to know that he had saved the lives of four very sick individuals. They also told us of his unrealized plans to be with his long time love when she returned to Illinois, and they shared the fact that he had a passion for his nieces, fishing, Eric Clapton, and the Chicago Bears. He was apparently also quite handy around the house, and since he lived only a few miles from both of his sisters, they constantly called upon him. They told us that they still find themselves reaching for the phone whenever something pops up. But they also said that they are comforted by the fact that he lives on through others and that he has been "well placed." The organ donation counselor asked them if she could do anything for them, and their only response was, "Find good homes for our brother." I must admit that the pain that I felt as I read the letter was intertwined with guilt. There was guilt for the fact that their lives are so much emptier, and our lives are so much fuller. And there was guilt for the fact that I have lost my focus lately. After returning to work, I have found myself getting angry or annoyed with the irrelevant details of life: the guy in front of me is driving too slowly, that darned kid in fifth hour refuses to do his homework, I can't believe that the condo association is levying a special assessment, I can't believe that CD interest rates are so pathetically low, why is there so much crap on the kitchen counter, why can't Madison schedule the bronch on Wednesday, and why do these pants make my thighs look so big? Everything has been annoying me lately. In fact, when Doug asked me what was bothering me last night, I tersely responded, "My existence." I'm not completely sure what I meant by that statement, but I am still in the process of sorting through the emotions of the transplant experience, and I'm just tired. I think too much, and that is my downfall. Nevertheless, the letter today was a slap in the face for me. Hello, have you forgotten everything you learned during this experience? Quit sweating the small stuff, and start focusing on the important things in life. Savor the sweetness, and let the crap roll off of you. Crap sinks, crap floats, and I believe that it also slides—SO LET IT SLIDE. I have decided that human beings are ultimately very poor learners. We learn life lessons and we are forever changed, but then life moves forward, and we allow ourselves to get caught up in the trivial and irrelevant once again. And then we ignorantly bumble along until something slaps us upside the head. Well, I got my slap upside the head today in the form of a letter. God bless that family for their generosity never ceases.

10/14/03

Doug had a bronch today, and the news was good and bad. The good news is that Doug's airways are looking very good. His left anastomosis is completely healed, and his right bronchus (the one with the stent) looks significantly better than it did during his last bronch. The doctor did not see any signs of Aspergillus, but he will wait on the cultures of the bronchial lavage before discontinuing the IV's.

The bad news is that Doug's blood test showed a white blood cell count of only 1,000. The normal range is 3,500-10,500. So the poor guy's immune system is severely compromised, and he is once again an inpatient at Madison. The doctors don't know what is causing this, but the two leading suspects are a virus or his anti-rejection med. They have run a blood test for CMV (a common tx virus), and they have done blood cultures and a CT scan. We should have some answers tomorrow, but in the meantime, they are stopping his Mycophenolate (rejection med) and putting him on an IV to increase his white cells. Because his immune system is so compromised, he is in isolation. No one is supposed to enter his room without washing their hands and wearing a mask.

Doug is feeling reasonably well, but he is scared. If his tests are positive for CMV, the doctor said that it will require IV's that can last anywhere from a week to several months. Since he has been on the anti-fungal IV's for four months, he is worried that he will once again be chained to the IV pole. We are hoping and praying that the low count is just a rejection med issue. Could we be so lucky?

I have returned home, and I will go back to work tomorrow. I called him when I got back home this evening, and I'm already feeling guilty that he is alone. I would give anything to be with him, but it doesn't make sense to use more sick time when tomorrow is just going to involve sitting around waiting for the doctor's news. I'm sure that it will be difficult to concentrate at work, and it is highly likely that the first teenager to work my nerves will lose an appendage, but that's why we have school nurses.

I would again appreciate your thoughts and prayers as we move forward through our next unknown. My mind is in a whirlwind again, and I'm thinking too much. I have been having a recurrent dream lately, and I have been thinking a lot about it today. I haven't given the dream much thought until today because I can't even figure out my conscious life. But since I had nothing but time while waiting during Doug's bronch, I gave the dream some thought, and I think that I have figured it out. The dream is very simple: I am in a stark white room with a card table that is filled with puzzle pieces that are all the same color. I try to do the puzzle, and just when I find some pieces that go together, a faceless man always enters the room and dumps more pieces on the table. It is at that point that I always wake up. I decided today that the puzzle represents the past six months of my life. I have been trying desperately to process all of my experiences and emotions and somehow make them fit together: my memory of the long ride to the hospital on the day of his transplant, saying good-bye to him before he entered the operating room, waiting for eight hours during his surgery, seeing him struggle for his life on the vent, watching the vent be removed, watching him take his first steps, being released from the hospital, dealing with Prednisone induced mood swings, fighting with doctors, battling depression, living with constant uncertainty, enduring endless bronchs, and receiving the donor letter. These are just a few of the puzzle pieces that I have to put together to find some sort of emotional peace. But the pieces just don't seem to fit together, and when I am finally able to find a connection, another piece is added. Today's new battle is just another puzzle piece. I imagine that if I have this dream again tonight, the faceless bastard will dump a mother load of puzzle pieces on my table. I think that I'm going to tell him to f...k off. I'll keep you posted.

10/15/03

I just spoke to Doug, and all of his blood work has come back clean. There is no sign of a bacterial infection, and there is no sign of CMV. His bronchial lavage also came back clean—no sign of Aspergillus or CMV in his lungs. Because the lung cultures came back clean, Doug has finally taken off of the anti-fungal IV. Ah, did you just hear that? That was my big sigh of relief. Doug's white blood cell count was still at 1,000 this morning, and he is still running intermittent fevers. The doctor did tell him that if the CMV test were to come back negative, they would probably place the blame for his current problems on his two anti-fungal meds and his rejection med (Mycophenolate). Once his WBC count has stabilized, they will resume the anti-fungal oral med and the rejection med, but the IV anti-fungal is finally history!

Since it has been a while since I have had a story of the medically ridiculous, I'll brighten your evening with my current annoyances. To begin, I received a call from Doug asking me if I had told the resident to withhold his IV anti-fungal yesterday after the bronch. I told him that I had not, and then relayed that the resident and I had only discussed the possibility of withholding his rejection med. It seems that the nurses were refusing to give Doug his IV because the resident had noted that I had told him to hold it. Umm, hello? First, we didn't discuss the IV anti-fungal, and secondly, when did I become a doctor? If I had told the resident to stick a flaming hot poker up Doug's orifice, would he have written orders to do so? Anyway, I later received a message from Doug's nurse stating that he needed to talk to me about the IV issue. When I called the unit, the unit coordinator told me that everything was squared away and that Doug would get the IV. But he then asked why I had told the resident to hold the IV. Oh, Jesus,

Mary, Joseph, and other assorted biblical characters, I DIDN'T TELL HIM TO HOLD ANYTHING. I then told him that if there were a question about whether or not he should be given the IV, then perhaps they should page the damn doctor instead of asking me. When I talked to Doug a few hours later, he still had not received the med, and his nurse still wanted to talk to me. So I had the pleasure of telling the nurse that I did not discontinue the med, and I also told him that if I HAD told the resident to do so, he should have talked to the attending about the issue. I AM NOT A DOCTOR, FOR THE LOVE OF GOD. I have been praying for the day when Madison would finally start listening to us, but this is ridiculous. I can apparently now write medical orders—wow, and I didn't even have to go through the hassle of going to med school.

Meanwhile, Doug will stay in the hospital until his white blood cell counts returns to at least 3,000. The IV therapy that they are using to stimulate to cell growth will take a minimum of three days, so we are looking at Friday as the earliest time for his release. I will stay at home and work until Friday and then head for Madison immediately after school. Doug doesn't want me to come over because he is concerned about my mental and physical health and doesn't want me driving after working all day. In all honesty, I think that he is just concerned that I might lose my last shred of sanity and hurt someone at the hospital—smart man.

10/16/03

Doug's fevers began to creep up again last night (101.5), he has had some vomiting spells, and his white blood cell count has now dropped to 900. He spoke with his doctor at 10:00 a.m. this morning, and he was told that they were going to start IV antibiotics since they are now suspecting something bacterial in nature. But as of 3:00 p.m., he had yet to receive any antibiotics, and to make matters worse, none had even been ordered. Since my fuse is so short, I called the transplant administrator, and we essentially agreed to disagree. She reduced my frustrations down to the following:

1. Doug didn't ask the right questions. She actually told me that the

doctors give patients as little information as possible because they find that most patients just don't want to know or just don't understand.

2. I am frustrated because I'm not in Madison, and I cannot advocate for him as I typically do.

She said that she would investigate the anti-fungal incident from yesterday and that she would also investigate the delay in starting the antibiotics today. But honestly, does it even matter?

Around 5:00 p.m., the infectious disease doctors came by, and they finally made an executive decision to put him on three IV antibiotics and restart all of the anti-fungals. Yes, these are the same anti-fungals that were discontinued yesterday because they lower the white blood cell count. The doctor said that it was a precaution to keep the Aspergillus from resurfacing, but I don't know what that will mean for his white blood cell count.

I am beyond frustrated and beyond tired. The tears of frustration and fear seem to come in waves tonight, and I told Doug that I simply can't battle them anymore. So I'm done. In fact, I am going to take a break from writing to all of you for a while. If something catastrophic occurs, I will let you know. Otherwise, I need a break. Expelling my emotions through this medium used to be helpful, but now it is just sickening to rehash everything at the end of the day—and please don't write me to tell me that I need to see a counselor. I'm not broken.

10/26/03

I figured that it was about time to come out of hiding and give everyone an update on Doug. First, I want to thank everyone who wrote such encouraging and supportive notes last week. The notes and your kindness were tremendously appreciated, and I apologize for not responding. I have shared just about every emotion that I have experienced since Doug's transplant, and I just needed some time to step away from everyone. I appreciate your indulgence, and I think that I am ready to return to the land of the living.

Doug was released from the hospital last Monday evening, and he came home on two IV's. He is on an antibiotic for the E-Coli that was found in his bloodstream, and he is once again on the IV for

Aspergillus. He will end the antibiotic on Friday, and he will end the IV anti-fungal when they get the blood level from his oral med. If the blood level is therapeutic, they will discontinue the IV that he has been on for nearly five months. So we are praying with the passion of twenty possessed monks that he can be IV free in about ten days. I can't tell you what that will mean to both of us. After three PICC line infections, four PICC lines, six inpatient stays, and an IV pole that has become part of our living room decor, we are beyond sick of IV's and everything that goes with them.

Doug and I are doing fairly well. In all honesty, last week was one of the most stressful weeks since his transplant. I won't bore you with all of the sordid details, but we had another bundle of battles. In fact, I engaged in three very heated discussions with the transplant administrator, a resident, and an infectious disease doctor. There were a number of times in which I was listening to myself talk during these heated exchanges, and I couldn't help marveling at the stranger who now inhabits my psyche. I have changed tremendously. I have become much more aggressive and assertive, which is good, but I have also become very bitter and angry. Doug told me the other day that he misses the old Dana. He told me that I don't smile or laugh like I used to, and unfortunately, he is right. I have lost a bit of the wonder and awe that I experienced at the onset of Doug's transplant. We are still grateful for the tremendous blessing of Doug's new lungs, but the frustration of the past few months has clouded much of the joy. And of course, I feel guilty about that. I just don't want to feel anymore.

11/03/03

During the past week or so Doug had developed a bit of a wheeze, and over the weekend it turned into a sound that resembled a collection of tortured souls. Doug and I have begun to affectionately refer to his stent (the constant source of his intermittent wheeze) as Purgatory. "Wow, it's an active day in Purgatory." Anyway, Purgatory became quite active in the middle of the night on Sunday, and neither one of us slept very much. I took his pulse ox before I left for work, and his O2 saturation had dropped to 94 percent, and his pulse was 110. We both agreed that he needed to call Madison to move up his November 11th bronch.

After working for an hour and in the midst of a tremendously teachable moment, Doug called and said that Madison wanted him there immediately. He was told that the surgeon would bronch him after he completed his current case. Doug also calmly mentioned to me that "he was having some trouble breathing." I called out to my biblical characters, flew out the door, and drove Doug to Madison.

We arrived at 10:00 a.m., and they took us back to the surgical cube. To make a very long story short, Doug did not go into the operating room until 6:30 that evening. The doctor was ready long before that, but there were no operating rooms available because of previously scheduled surgeries and trauma cases. After they finally took him, I normally wait anywhere between twenty to sixty minutes to hear the results of Doug's bronchs. But when 8:00 rolled around, the adrenaline started to pulsate with the ferocity of a severed artery. Finally, the doctor appeared about 8:15 and announced, "Boy, that was a tour de force." He handed me a picture and then proceeded to explain that his stent was 100 percent occluded. It was so occluded that the flexible bronch wouldn't remove the junk, and they had to switch to a rigid bronch.

I finally got to see Doug sometime after 9:00, and the poor guy kept puking from the anesthesia—not an easy task when you haven't eaten in over twenty four hours. He was extremely loopy, but he was adamant that he wanted to go home. The doctor said that there was no need to keep him, and so we drove home at 10:00 in Wisconsin's version of a monsoon. It was probably a stupid move because I was beyond exhausted, and I found that focusing on the road was a major challenge. Doug was so drugged that I don't even think he noticed the times that I drifted a little too close to the shoulder of the road. We did make it home without becoming organ donors, and I decided to take a sick day this morning. I felt like I had been beaten with a thousand bronchoscopes, and the thought of managing teenagers was just too much. I thought about "toughing it out," but I decided that "screw toughing it out" was a much better philosophy for the day.

11/04/03

As you may or may not remember, Doug and I have been waiting oh so patiently for the results of his Voriconazole level. Now remember class, if the level is therapeutic, Doug gets to end the IV that he has been on for the past five months. His coordinator called this evening and reluctantly told us that there was a mix up on the blood draw. It seems that our local hospital sent the sample as an Itraconazole test instead of a Voriconazole test. As a result, the blood test has to be redone, and we have to wait another two weeks for the results.

We were again stunned by our seemingly endless chain of bad luck. I told the coordinator that we just can't seem to catch a break. She agreed and then told me that when the results came across her desk, she immediately thought, "How am I going to tell them this?" Well, I guess you just open your mouth and let the fecal matter flow. Fly feces, fly. Needless to say, Doug and I are beyond disappointed, and we have already had a good frustrated cry—it didn't really help. Now we just look like prize fighters with swollen eyes.

11/17/03

Doug found out today that his oral anti-fungal drug is indeed at a therapeutic level. This means that he does not have to restart the IV anti-fungals unless his bronchs show something funky in the future. To celebrate, I busted a move and did a no more IV's dance. If you would like to participate in my fun, just picture a Michael Jackson moon walk being done by a white girl...oh wait, Michael Jackson is a white girl. And just so you know, I omitted the crotch grabbing part.

11/23/03

It is once again that festive holiday season, and as Thanksgiving approaches, it is a good time to reflect upon those things for which we are grateful. I would like to share my gratitude list with you, and I encourage you to think about the little things in your life that make your existence so extra special.

1. Profanity: I have developed a profound sense of gratitude this

year for every profane word in the English language. My lewd vocabulary has helped me express my feelings in a way that Hallmark never could.

2. Lemons: I think that we have all heard the expression that encourages us to make lemonade when life hands us lemons. That's good advice, but ladies, did you know that lemons can also be used to bleach your mustache?

3. Michael Jackson: He's one of the few people that I can look at and honestly say, "Yes, yes, I'm prettier than he is."

4. Computers: They have taught me humility. Whenever I turn one on, I am reminded that I am not really all that smart. They also allow me to experience more gratitude for my ability to use profanity.

5. CNN Headline News: It's the only channel where I can to listen to a reporter, watch news footage, read the crawl at the bottom of the screen, and see the date, time, weather forecast, and sports scores all at the same time. But since it can be so overwhelming, it makes me feel a lot less guilty about my binge drinking and crack habit. "I just need something to take the edge off. I just watched CNN Headline News for God's sake."

6. Algebra Class: It made me believe in my psychic powers. I predicted as a freshman in high school that I would never have any use for the class. Yeah Miss Cleo, you're not the only one who can predict the future.

7. The Transplant Team: Refer back to #1.

8. God's Wisdom: I'm grateful that God understood that putting horns on a cat would have been a very bad idea. I think we can all agree that those darn claws hurt enough—adding horns to the mixture would have been supremely intolerable.

9. Spandex: It has helped my body image tremendously. Sure, I look like a sausage stuffed too tightly into its casing, but even the thin girls look like they're ready to be served up with a side of eggs. I take great comfort in that.

10. Fungus: I have learned to appreciate the difference between a good fungus and a bad fungus. Mushrooms on my pizza are very good things, but a fungus in my husband's lungs is a very bad thing.

Remember class, if your fungus cannot be used as a pizza topping, it's just not a good fungus.

11/25/03

Doug had another bronch today, and he is once again the proud father of another snot baby. He and his stent have been quite the prolifically fertile pair, but let me just say that those damn snot babies are good for nothing. They offer no unconditional love—they just get snotty and decide to block an airway. Since his airway has finally healed, the doctor thinks that his body is now trying to naturally wash the stent out. It's a foreign object, and since his body doesn't want it there...voila...snot. I really love the body's approach. I don't like you—I'm going to snot you out. You truly have to appreciate the body's philosophy. There's no indecision, no ethical debate, and no second chances—there's just snot.

We did talk to the doctor about removing the stent, but he and the head surgeon are still debating the issue. Apparently, they are engaged in some sort of medical forensics competition. Fine, you can debate and then debate some more, but at some point we need a winner, boys.

And of course, we did have a moment of comedic tragedy. When the doctor came in to see Doug before his surgery, he asked, "Where are we at with the Caspofungin (anti-fungal IV)?" Doug and I looked at one another quizzically, and I stifled a chuckle. Doug said, "Umm, I've been off of that for about three weeks." "Oh great," said the doctor. It seems that he forgot that he personally made the decision to discontinue it. If I were a lung, I would have created a little snot and washed him out of the room!

12/19/03

As the snow begins to fall and the barren trees silhouette the wintry sky, the final chapter of 2003 is being composed. And while the pages of our year were filled with unforgettable and challenging experiences, every page resonated with hope—the belief that each new day held the promise of something better. Throughout the days of this past year, Doug and I have been sustained and nurtured by hope. We learned that hope is why we get out of bed in the morning. Hope is why we battle his disease and dare to love one another. Hope is what allows us to believe that there is always the possibility that we just might be triumphant no matter what the odds. It is the spirit that enables us to endure all of life's challenges. A cancer patient once said to her doctor, "You can take my hair, but don't you dare take my hope. It's all I have." So finish life's race, fight the battle; believe in the miracle—hope is by your side. Doug and I would like to wish you a very merry Christmas or a very happy Hanukkah, and we pray that the New Year will bring you abundant joy and health.

1/06/04

Doug celebrated a bronchial anniversary today by having his 25th bronch since his transplant. That's a SILVER anniversary, people—you know, like the silver gifts that you should be sending him! He is currently celebrating the big day by sleeping in the lovely and gentle land of sweet dreams and Versed (the sedative used during bronchs). For the past five months, the transplant surgeons have been doing his bronchs, but today we returned to the pulmonologist after growing very weary of operating rooms, anesthesiologists, and general anesthesia for simple and routine bronchs. Doug requested the return to the pulmonologist, and the tx team saw no reason to deny his wishes. Things went smoothly, and as usual, Doug gave birth to yet another delightfully rambunctious snot baby. In fact, the doctor said that he had to engage in a bit of tug of war with the little bugger because it did not want to surrender its bronchial home. So there was nothing new there. But the pulmonologist did discuss several interesting things with us...well, with me since Doug was virtually comatose. He told me the following:

1. He believes that Doug should not have been going under general anesthesia for his previous bronchs. Hmm, that's an interesting thought. Doug and I have been saying the same thing for the past few months, but we must now file that thought in the "oh, well" category.

2. He told me that the tx surgeons had prescribed the wrong med

to eliminate the snot babies. Doug had been doing a nebulized drug (Pulmozyme) twice a day, but the pulmonologist said that this would do little to break down the secretions. He started talking about the lack of DNA in Doug's secretions, and then I basically got lost and utterly confused and started daydreaming. At any rate, Doug's nebulized med has been discontinued, and he has now been started on Zithromax (to aide in the mucous/inflammation cycle) and Guaifenesin (an expectorant). As a side note, we were told that the damn Guaifenesin is no longer available as a prescription, and it will cost about $100 a month. I have made jokes about the snot babies, but now I feel like I'm buying baby formula for the little bastards.

3. He told us that Doug has a dysfunctional right diaphragm that compounds the stent and mucous issue. Hmm, that was news to us. Apparently, it is not uncommon for a nerve to be cut during the tx surgery that damages the diaphragm's ability to function properly. Remarkably, they don't consider this to be a serious problem, but it does make it more difficult for Doug to clear the secretions that his bronchus is generating due to the stent. Doug's coordinator told us that he has likely had this issue since his surgery, but she said that the physicians typically don't share this kind of information with her. When she talked to the tx surgeon about it, he said, "I know about the diaphragm, but part of it still works." I guess that would be like my sanity—part of it still exists.

4. He believes that it is time to take out the stent. So he will meet with the transplant surgeon and Doug's coordinator, and they will huddle together like a football team and come up with a play. Everyone agrees that Doug's airways are looking very healthy, and everyone concurs that the stent needs to go. The only question remaining is when. And whether it is a week from today or two to three months down the road, the stent will come out, and the transplant team will be soon be able to celebrate the play by rejoicing in the proverbial transplant end zone. And perhaps, just maybe, Doug and I will sprint down to that transplant end zone and give each one of them a quick pat on the butt and spike that stent like nobody's business.

2/03/04

It is with tremendous joy that I announce to you that Doug's stent has been given its proverbial pink slip. It's done...relieved of its duty...retiring...moving to Florida...looking to play some Canasta and Shuffleboard in the stent community center. After seven months of supporting Doug's bronchus and making snot babies like a possessed rabbit, it is time to exit stage right—or would that be exit bronchus right? Our stent friend has served Doug well, but we are very eager to bid it a very fond adieu. Careful there, my little stent, don't let the operating room doors hit you in the stent ass as you leave.

Doug had a CT scan last Friday, and today we were told that his stented bronchus looks "anatomically good." That's the transplant surgeon's romantic way of saying that he is ready to remove the stent. As a result, Doug will have the bronchial retirement party either next week or the following week. I will let you know when we have a date, and I look forward to letting you know that the stent has moved on to bigger and better things.

2/04/04

I received an email today in which I was asked if I could give a glimpse of how our lives have changed since Doug's tx. I'm happy to oblige, and while our life is not perfect, I hope that our experience will encourage anyone who is uncertain about the transplant journey and illuminate those who are just curious.

In the six month period before his tx, Doug's lung function dipped to a paltry 16%. Toward the end of his wait, he was using O2 twenty-four hours a day, and his breathing had become so labored that he began to use Xanax to reduce the sensation of being smothered. Life had been reduced to a test of mental and physical endurance. Simple tasks like showering, bending over to tie his shoes, walking from the car to a store, and climbing a flight of stairs were major physical challenges. Laughing became impossible, as it would only lead to uncontrollable coughing spells. Doug also began to suffer from routine bouts of hemoptysis (coughing up blood), and each bout seemed to get progressively worse. He was transported to a hospital by ambulance twice when his hemoptysis became severe. Lung infections became routine, and his lungs crackled and groaned under the weight of the constant infections. Doug found himself with a PICC line and IV antibiotics every few months, and doctor's visits became as common as trips to the grocery store.

Doug's days were reduced to regimented medical routines. He would get up and take a handful of pills, nebulize Pulmicort and Pulmozyme, struggle to breathe during his shower, use the Vest and Flutter while struggling not to vomit because of the intense coughing, and then finally inhale the antibiotic du jour. In the afternoon, he exercised on the treadmill, lifted weights, and repeated his chest PT. Then in the evening, Doug would repeat his morning routing of chest PT, meds, and nebs. But despite all of his effort, his health continued to deteriorate. He slowly began to lose his freedom, he became chained to our home, and he had to rely on others to help him through his days. His existence became a daily struggle, and every day was reduced to primal survival.

Immediately after his transplant, Doug's new lungs were eerily silent, and he could breathe without thought or effort. As you know, Doug has had numerous complications, but our path is getting smoother, and the Doug who exists today bears no resemblance to the Doug of ten months ago. He can, quite simply, do anything he wants. The physical chains that once bound him are gone. He is a free man, and he loves his life and his freedom. We have no regrets, and although our future will never be certain, we are relishing the sweet nectar of this transplant. It is a pure miracle, and words cannot capture the dramatic change.

Doug's current routine is in stark contrast with his daily routine of ten months ago. Each day, we are awoken by our chamber maids just as the sun begins to peak through the curtains. We then listen to classical music while waiting for our butler to serve us breakfast in bed. Sometimes, Doug will run a quick mile or two around the estate before breakfast, and then we saunter off to the spa...oh, wait...that isn't our life. I sometimes get caught up in my royal family delusion. Dana and Doug—queen and king. The truth be told, we are actually nothing more than village idiots who can only aspire to greatness.

In all seriousness, I can relate Doug's routine in just a few sentences. He gets up, takes six pills, takes a shower, does a home pulmonary function test, takes his temperature and blood pressure, and is on his merry way to his job at Barnes and Noble. Of course in my mind, he heads off to the royal palace to sit upon the throne, but let's get back to reality. In the afternoon, he takes his vitamins and exercises, and in the evening, he takes seven pills. That's it, people. There is no more hemoptysis, no more O2, no Vest or Flutter, no Pulmozyme, no more vomit coughs, and no more breathlessness. And most importantly, he can laugh again. In fact, we are both laughing again. I have little doubt that I would be standing at the foot of my husband's grave if it were not for this miracle. We have been given a second chance. Life is good, and we owe it all to a little thing called a double lung transplant.

2/09/04

For those of you who are inclined to seek divine aid, Doug and I would like to ask you to say a prayer or two for him as he has his stent removed on Tuesday. The doctors feel that his bronchus is strong enough to support itself, but there are no guarantees. To quote one of the transplant surgeons, "You know, we could remove that stent, and that airway could just collapse on itself. If that happens, there is going to be a collective gasp, and we are going to have to move very quickly." Prayers? People, do I hear those prayers? Doug's bronchus is like a child who comes home after graduating from college. There are a number of unresolved questions: Are you going to be able to support yourself, or am I going to have to continue supporting your sorry ass? At least stents can't talk back. The doctors also mentioned that the removal might be a bit bloody since the stent has become embedded in the tissue. Hmm, there's yet another comforting thought. I'll update you on Tuesday.

2/10/04

Our day began at 4:30 a.m., and I would just like to mention that this is an extremely dark time of the day. I didn't know this before, but I find 4:30 in the morning to be a supremely unpleasant time. You can file this tidbit under the 101 things that you never knew about Dana. At any rate, we have a stent story to tell. It's really quite simple—the bastard stent put up a fight, but it came out without causing a scene, and the airway is as stiff as a board. "The airway looks really good. This couldn't have gone better. Doug is one lucky man. I couldn't have predicted such a positive end to this problem. This was a very grave situation for seven months, but we are finally out of the woods." By the way, those are the surgeon's words—email sound bites for your reading pleasure. Those are very lovely words, but we discovered some other very interesting facts today. First, we were told that Doug is lucky to be alive. It seems that most people who have had Doug's problem are currently six feet under. Hmm, we knew that the situation was serious, but we had no idea that we should have been hanging out at church and chapel to pre-plan Doug's funeral. Secondly, after his procedure today, we discovered that they had banked blood for him and shaved his chest in case of a major stent disaster. He was sitting in his bed after the surgery, and his gown had slipped off of his shoulders. I was staring at him and wondering why he suddenly looked so "boyish." It finally dawned on me that he was missing his chest hair. I can be so ridiculously obtuse at times. We were a little shocked that they had prepared him to be cut open in an emergency. While we were contemplating that frightening scenario, Doug looked at me and said, "Oh God, how far down did they shave me?" He couldn't bear to look at the potential repeat of the Brazilian shave of his transplant days, so I did the honors. "The rain forest of Rio de Janeiro has not been cut down, Doug. All is well." That was probably way too much information, but it was such a moment of comic relief that I just felt compelled to share it with you. In spite of the shaving giggles, this was a very emotional day. Today reminded me of the day that his breathing tube was pulled after his transplant. That was such a huge milestone in his journey, and the removal of the stent is the second huge milestone. The past nine months have been absolutely hellacious, and we finally feel like we have concluded this part of the race. We have won this particular battle. There will inevitably be others, but this was one big win, people. There is an odd combination of relief, joy, and supreme exhaustion. This has been a huge physical and emotional battle, and the past several months have challenged us to our absolute limits. We have been holding our breath for too long, and now we can finally breathe again. Well, I have been able to breathe well all along. It's Doug who has occasionally found the breathing process to be a bit of a challenge. But that is now just another lovely memory of the transplant process.

So we have reached the end of the Aspergillus/stent story, and the conclusion is a happy one. What do you do when your dream comes true? You step back, savor it, catalogue it, and move forward, for this is not the end of the story. It's only the beginning. God bless all of you, and Doug and I thank you from the bottom of our hearts for your endless prayers and support.

3/02/04

Doug had a bronch today to check his previously stented bronchus. The bronchus looked perfect, and the transplant surgeon, who isn't prone to smiling, grinned and said, "The bronchus couldn't look better. It looks like this is the end of the story." Well, there you have it—the end of the story, my friends. It has been one heck of a year, and it has been one heck of a story. So what have I learned from this story? Let me share a few things with you:

1. Transplantation is not good for my face. I haven't looked good for a year! I'm so damn tired.

2. Anesthesia eliminates all shreds of intelligence, rational thought, and humor. Doug just isn't very fun after surgery.

3. I really like to swear when I get angry. I'm certain that I could beat even the best sailors and truckers in a swearing contest.

4. Driving to Madison is slightly more entertaining than watching the dust slowly collect on the coffee table in the family room.

5. Hospitals don't smell good.

6. Hospital food doesn't smell good either. I won't even comment on the taste.

7. Waiting rooms aren't as charming as they could be, and waiting room chairs leave a lot to be desired. I never knew how many pain receptors the human butt has.

8. Hospital art isn't art. Did they get a special deal at the starving artists' sale at the local Marriott?

9. Transplant surgeons don't speak English. Is it Latin? Have I been exposed to secondhand amnesia? I'm just never sure what they're trying to tell me.

10. Using the shampoo that the hospital provides leaves your hair dull, limp, and lifeless. Honestly, how good can a non-rinse shampoo be?

11. Vomit buckets should come in a variety of colors. Vomit always comes in a variety of colors, so shouldn't the apparatus that catches it be just as colorful?

12. You know that you have spent too much time in the hospital when you start to bond with the cleaning crew.

13. Hospitals run on Latin American time. Three o'clock actually means sometime between three and nine.

14. Nurses are angels on Earth.

15. I'm grateful that there are human beings on this Earth who are masochistic enough to endure medical school and the insane schedule of a doctor.

16. Doug and I are stronger than I ever imagined. And despite the odds against him, the little bastard is still alive. And as for me, I'm still standing by his side, and I'm still ready to do battle when and if necessary. But given a choice, I would rather go to bed and rest for a while.

If one person falls, the other can reach out and help. But people who are alone when they fall are in real trouble.

—Ecclesiastes 4:10 (NLT)

Life on an Online Support Group

The following writings are posts that Doug and I contributed to Cystic-L, one of our online support groups. They represent the seriousness and the levity of living with cystic fibrosis.

Doug wrote the following post in response to a woman who was contemplating suicide. She had lost all of her hope, and she was giving serious consideration to stopping all of her medication.

I'm glad you wrote your post on Sunday. I think it probably threw many people for a loop, but the fact of the matter is that many people on this list have had similar thoughts. And at this point in your life, having people say, "Just hang in there" doesn't really work. So I'm afraid to say, there are no rose colored words that will magically ignite you to become a new person in this particular post. Quite frankly, I really don't think one line quotes transmitted through email really do much anyway. I'm thirty-seven years old, and in 1984 I went through the same struggle that you're going through now. I was just out of high school, had no plans, no meaning and no purpose to my life, and my health was going down hill. I didn't really think beyond two or three months. I never imagined I would be alive to see the year 2000. That was a very difficult time for me, filled with darkness, anger, confusion, and the harsh recognition of how impoverished my life really was. In retrospect, I can see that what I was dealing with and confronting was time itself and the uncertainty of time. As you already know, the most difficult thing for anyone who has a terminal illness is figuring out how to deal with the many uncertainties which plague our day-to-day life. We are uncertain about what course our health will take, how our finances will do, how our family and friends will react, etc., etc., etc. I wish I could give you a simple code or principle, or simply say, "Read this book; it will change your life!" But I'm not Oprah, so I can't. The reality is that there is no simple solution to what you are experiencing. I can tell you from my own experience that getting yourself out of the abyss you're in will be very hard, draining, and exhausting. There is no easy solution. There is no one right way. There is no set of ten rules for life that I can post here and change everything. You, and only you, know what you have gone through, how much energy you still have in you, and how much of your fighting spirit remains. The only thing that kept me going and kept me alive was deciding to accept any joy or excitement in life despite the pains and agonies of a terminal illness. I decided to accept the good and the bad of what my life would bring. Have you seen Vanilla Sky? I think it was the best movie of 2001. One of the themes of this movie is making oneself accept the good and the bad in life together; to accept the "sweet and sour" in life. The best moment of the film is when Tom Cruise sees Penelope Cruz on the roof of the building for the last time. It is sad because he has to say good-bye to his dream of a perfect life, complete acceptance, and total unconditional love. He isn't saying good-bye to her; he is saying good-bye to his dreams and his fantasies about what his life should be. He then made the biggest decision he's ever made and accepted life despite the pain, loneliness, and numerous moments of meaninglessness. So this is what it boils down to: will you accept the joys and hopes of life even if that means that you must also accept the pain and disappointment that comes with it? This is your decision, and only you know what your threshold is and how much you want to endure. It isn't fair that you should have to make this decision, but it is the reality you are in right now. I know because I've been there too. As the great philosopher Anna Nicole Smith says, "Shit Happens. Then instead of dying, you live, and then more shit happens." I do wish you well. Please keep everyone here posted on what is going on with you.

I wrote this post in response to a man who was wondering if he would ever be able to establish a relationship with a woman. He didn't think that anyone would ever be able to see beyond his illness to love him.

My name is Dana, and I am married to Doug. I was touched by your postings about the challenges of establishing and maintaining relationships while dealing with a serious illness. They reminded me of when my husband and I first started dating. When I first found out that he had CF, I knew very little about the disease. So I made a trip to the library to read all about it. My first response was, "Holy crap, what am I getting myself into?" Since Doug had told me that he had CF on our fourth date, I had already developed a slight fondness for him. I thought long and hard about the situation, and I ultimately decided that if I stopped dating him solely because of his illness, I would be a shallow schmuck. And while I can handle being a schmuck, I certainly can't handle being shallow. So we forged ahead, and gradually my fondness for him turned to love. I know that Doug often wondered about the fairness of asking a young and healthy woman to accept the burden of living with CF. But we persevered, and we have now been married almost seven years. There have been some challenges, some low points, and some self-pity, but I have never regretted my decision to get involved with someone who has a serious illness. I understand that there are some people who are unwilling or unable to deal with a serious illness, but there are so many who are. If and when you find someone who wants to be with you, do not fight it. Be open to the possibility of love and accept the fact that someone is willing to love you. No one should have to face this disease alone, and no one should be alone because of this disease. You DO deserve to be loved. And while embracing a relationship that involves a serious illness is difficult, living a full and rich life is about accepting and welcoming challenge. What have you learned from something that was easy? Always remember that no one, healthy or ill, is guaranteed tomorrow. In the immortal words of Hank Williams, "NO ONE will get out of this world alive." We are all destined to the same fate, and we should all be destined to experience a little bit of love while we are here. You may not meet your soul mate or get married, but please make sure that you do not rob someone of the experience of loving you. Don't push people away because you think that you will protect them by doing so. Cystic fibrosis may rob you of your breath, but don't let it rob you of your ability to give and receive love. I absolutely hate CF, but it has given me a perspective for which I will be eternally grateful. I see the beauty of the small and simple things in life, and I value family and friends and time spent with them like never before. So boys, go out and find some nice girls....

Life on an online support groups always includes periods of dissention, disagreements, and fighting. I wrote the following post during a particular period in which the bickering and pettiness were becoming overwhelming.

It has always been very interesting to read the posts and ride the waves at Cystic-L: "No one responds to me. Please stop responding to me. I need advice. Quit sending me advice. I'm so grateful for the support on this list. No one supports me." I think you get the picture! I have a lot of opinions, and I can never resist an opportunity to put in my two cents. Actually, I usually have so much to say that maybe I should put it on my credit card! Anyway, in regard to dealing with one another on this list, I think we all need to remember that the majority of people are very supportive and do what they can. And yes, there are times when we all drop the ball, ignore the ball, or throw the ball a little too hard—I like ball analogies. So here are my pearls of wisdom for the day: accept the support that is given and be grateful for it; when the list disappoints, be forgiving and move forward with the recognition that this is a list full of imperfect people. Most of us here have faulty genes, lungs, pancreases, livers, etc., so why do we think that our responses and emotions will always be perfect? Yes, we all sometimes need emotional enzymes to keep the crap from shooting from our mouths, but this is a good list, and I will always be grateful for the good, the bad, the ugly, the rambling, the ridiculous, and the occasional spice of a flame.

Doug wrote this post in response to a woman who had written that she was living in a constant state of fear because of CF. She stated her feelings in a simple and short line that completely captured the most basic and primal feeling of anyone who faces an illness: "I'm afraid." Doug was also at a low point in his life. He had recently been placed on the transplant list, and he was afraid that he was running out of time and energy. He was still battling CF with all of his might, but the physical and emotional battle was becoming progressively difficult.

Well, let's see, I woke up at 4:00 in the morning coughing up a little blood, and I am sitting here now listening to Beethoven and looking out my window at the Siberian frozen tundra that Milwaukee, Wisconsin has now become. What better time to reply to the "Afraid" post from a couple days ago! Everyone who has a life threatening illness goes through an intense period of being afraid; that is completely normal. But simply because it's normal doesn't make it any easier. About ten years ago, I was at my doctor's office, and I had the opportunity to look at my PFT (pulmonary function test) numbers. I remember calculating that I would be dead in four or five years if my decline continued to progress at a constant rate. At that moment, my world just stopped, and I was no longer part of it. I just sat there looking at the numbers on the sheets of computer paper, and I came to the full realization of what those numbers meant for me. I was simply horrified. It didn't matter what I would accomplish in the future because those numbers would eventually catch up to me and kill me. And there have been many times, especially before I got married, when I was living alone that I would cough up blood. I lived in downtown Milwaukee for several years, and I vividly remember coughing up blood one night and looking out my window at the city. I saw people walking and driving around, and I thought about how profoundly unfair it is that I (and all CF people) should have to deal with this. I knew that the average healthy person had no clue as to how life can be such an intense struggle. The raw fact of the matter is that nature is evil. As Thomas Hobbes said, "Life is short, nasty, and brutish." How true. Nature creates humans who require oxygen. So, we have these nice, warm, and moist lungs that are perfect for the task. But nature is also full of bacteria, and bacteria just love to take up residence in these warm lungs. And as a result of our genes, it is hard for us to fight off these bacteria, and we end up having these little bastards colonize and destroy our lungs. Now how stupid, convoluted, and mismanaged is that! So here we are, born into the world, full of life, and yet our own existence is threatened by bacterial entities that are also full of life. And, to make matters worse, we shouldn't even be close to other people with CF because of cross contamination. So we need to shield ourselves from bacteria and other people with CF. What a wonderful system nature has created! We are the recipients of this error, and one of the results of this is the constant underlying fear. Those of us who have fatal illnesses are forced to look into the horror of existence and see the reality of our own death staring back at us, unwavering and unmoved by our desires for a better life; a life free of suffering and pain. As harsh at it sounds, this is the reality that haunts every person with a major illness. Being afraid is completely normal, completely understandable, and completely justified. Okay, I'm done now; this has become a little too heavy even for me. I'm now going to turn off Beethoven, and turn on TV and watch the Telletubbies. Take Care!

Online support groups are not just filled with medical information and sadness. There are occasional moments of levity and silliness. I wrote this post on a day in which a member of the group had suggested that we introduce or reintroduce ourselves to the group. We sometimes got so caught up in the disease that we would forget that there were human beings behind the illness. This activity provided the perfect opportunity for us to remember that we are people with lives beyond CF. I decided to forego the traditional introduction and do something just a little different.

Doug and were wondering if we could be the official Village Idiots at Cystic-L? We are very qualified, and I'm quite certain that we won't disappoint. We have included our resume for your consideration:

Names: Doug & Dana.

Ages: 37 and 35. We are young enough to still be stupid, but old enough to recognize it.

Married: We joined forces almost eight years ago when we decided that two small brains would equal one normal brain. We knew that it was the only way that we could have a viable shot at survival in the world.

Professions: Bookseller at Barnes & Noble and Spanish Teacher. Yeah, somehow we are pulling it off! Please don't hold this against us. We still want to be your Idiots.

Children: Too dangerous to be responsible for youth, currently practicing on a cat. We are very pleased and relieved that he has those nine lives to fall back on.

Favorite food: Fish. It's good food for the brain.

Favorite color: Not sure how to answer. That's a tough question, and we're not really sure what you want here. Multiple-choice would have helped on this one.

Short-term goal: Being Village Idiots on Cystic-L. Really, we would be so honored.

Long-term goal: Becoming King and Queen on Cystic-L. It's not realistic, but we can dream. Also, we are trying to persuade the doctors to do a brain transplant along with the lungs. If this occurs, Doug will resign from his post immediately, and Dana will shoulder the burden by herself.

Seriously, Doug and I enjoy Cystic-L tremendously, and we have learned a great deal from all of you. Since things have been a little tense lately, we thought we might try a little levity through self-deprecation and humor. Stay healthy and laugh a little.

Dana & Doug, Village Idiots at Cystic-L

Is this too presumptuous? Should we wait for an official vote?

I wrote this post in response to a young woman who was thinking about having a baby. She was two years post transplant, and she was seeking advice and opinions about the risk that a pregnancy might pose to her health.

I have a couple of thoughts to share with you regarding your situation. First, as a woman married to a man with CF, I understand the reality of accepting a future without biological children. It is my reality, and I have come to accept it. Grieve the fact that you may never be able to have biological children, and then move forward and explore your options. It may very well be that you will never have children, and while that may not make you happy, it may be your reality. Again, grieve that void and focus on those things that bring joy to your life. I also have a perspective on this topic as a wife whose husband is awaiting a lung transplant. I understand that the wait for transplant is long, many don't survive the wait, and many don't survive the years following transplant. Given these odds and statistics, please focus on the fact that you are a very lucky and blessed woman. In my opinion, you have a responsibility to care for those new lungs to honor your donor and to honor all of those who never got the opportunity at a second chance. I can't tell you how much it pains me when I read stories about people who are careless about taking their meds or don't follow their center's advice and protocol. You have been given the greatest gift that anyone can receive TWICE. You were blessed with life on the day you were born, and you were blessed with a second life on the day you received your new lungs. Take care of those lungs, and take care of yourself. I wish you the very best.

I wrote this post in response to a woman who had stated that CF caregivers are caring individuals who always put their own needs behind the needs of others. She mentioned my name in the post because I had just spent several days sleeping in a chair during one of Doug's hospital stays. I love sarcasm, and I couldn't resist the temptation to unleash a little of the sardonic side of my personality.

Thanks so much for your post. It was nice to see my name mentioned next to the words kindness, endurance, and patience. I suppose that I could just let this go and bask in the flattery of your words, but alas, I must be honest. I secretly love hospitals and their many amenities. Yes, it is true. I just can't get enough of those vinyl hospital chairs. I truly love sleeping in them, and I love the way my flesh clings so fervently to the synthetic material. In fact, I tried to drag one down to the car during our last hospital visit, but security stopped me. I tried to fight the guy, but he was much stronger, and I had to relinquish the chair. I cried, but this guy was one heartless bastard. My tears and undeniable connection to the chair would not sway him.I love hospital food too. I love eating indistinguishable food products covered in indistinguishable sauces—it is truly an adventure in fun.

"What the hell is this?"

"I don't know, but let's dig in and eat it!"

"Hey, and what is that indistinguishable stain on the wall? It's an unusual shade of brown. Is it blood?"

"I don't know, but just keep your eye on it because it may be a living creature."

"And what is that smell? Oh dear God, let's not even go there."

So as you can see, I am not a good person. I just have a hospital fetish. Thanks for letting me get this off of my chest. It's a bit like a 12 step program: the first step is admitting that I have a problem. "Hi, my name is Dana, and I love hospitals."

Well, that's enough sarcasm for this evening. In all honesty, I was very flattered by your post, but I would honestly do anything for Doug. Sleeping in an uncomfortable vinyl chair surrounded by bad smells and bad stains and eating indistinguishable pooh on a platter is just what I do. And damn it, I do it well!

This post was written in response to a few individuals who were becoming disheartened and scared by Doug's constant post transplant "bumps." I was attempting to answer the question, "Is a transplant worth the struggle?"

I have been posting about Doug's transplant journey since day one to Cystic-L and Secondwind, and I just recently began to post to ConnColl. Why have I shared virtually every detail? For one simple reason: I wanted to keep family and friends updated, and I also wanted those who were considering a transplant to experience the journey in as much detail as possible. From the day that Doug was listed, I knew in my heart that I was supposed to share our journey, and I have not regretted my decision once. For those who are facing a transplant, I believe that it is important to know just how difficult the process is. My intention is not to scare, but rather to educate. Doug and I were so focused on the surgery and surviving the surgery that we gave little thought to the emotional battle and the almost guaranteed post transplant bumps. Every transplant is different, and each journey takes a different path, but in the end, the journey is always very difficult. But along with the difficulties, there is so much beauty and joy in this process. So for anyone who is wondering if a transplant is worth it, the answer is a hearty and enthusiastic, "ABSOLUTELY."

I wrote this post in response to a woman who had just lost a good friend to CF. She was angry at her friend's passing, and she was angry with God. She wondered how a loving God could allow a young and vibrant mother to die.

I did not know your friend, but I ache for everyone who suffers or dies at the hands of this cruel disease. I can offer you no real answers, comfort, or solace, but I can offer you my perspective on suffering, loss, and heartache. I do believe in God, and so that is where I find comfort. I believe that we live in a fallen world and that suffering is inevitable. In fact, we are promised a life full of suffering, but at the same time, God promises to be with us always. I am also comforted by the fact that Jesus felt the pain of loss and suffering in his life, so I believe that he weeps and hurts right along with us. But despite these core beliefs, I can tell you that God sometimes feels so distant, and I often feel very alone. When I watch my husband cough up blood or struggle to breathe, I get angry and I sometimes curse God. I cannot tell you the number of times that I have said to God in my most anguished CF moments, "Don't you do this to him." And while I ultimately don't believe that God is doing it to him, I don't know who else to yell at. And yes, despite my faith, I often wonder why life has to be this way. I am reminded of Jesus and his anguished cry to God as he suffered on the cross, "Why have you forsaken me?" I figure that if an anguished cry was good enough for Jesus, then it is good enough for me. There should be no shame in feeling angry, confused, and lost in the midst of losing a friend. Again, I am reminded that Jesus went away from his disciples and the crowds to be alone and grieve the death of his friend John the Baptist. I also believe that there is meaning in everything—happiness and suffering. I have struggled for years to try to comprehend the meaning, but I have decided that I will never completely understand the mystery of life. I know that I will in time, so I have learned to be content with that for the time being. In addition, I believe that there are two groups in this world: those who find solace in the belief of a higher being, and those who believe that they are ultimately on their own. I judge no one on their choice or belief, but I know that I personally find great solace in the fact that I believe that there is a benevolent creator who grieves with us and who will one day explain everything and welcome us to a place where there is no suffering. Without these beliefs, I can honestly tell you that I could not bear the heartache of cystic fibrosis. I believe that there is meaning in the struggle, and that one day, God will wipe away all of the tears. As I said in the beginning, no words or proclamation of faith can ease or explain the pain of loss, but as I have stated in some of my other posts, life is a collection of dark and difficult moments, and so we learn to savor the sweet hours in which our lives burst open and give us everything we have imagined (Michael Cunningham, *The Hours*). So, be angry, cry, and even yell at God. And when the sun rises tomorrow and life moves on, look for the beauty in the world and reflect upon and honor the brief but meaningful life of your friend.

In giving advice I advise you, be short.
—Horace

Life's Guiding Principles

1. Trust in God.
2. Life is a beautiful treasure. Savor its beauty.
3. Accept the fact that life is hard and inherently unfair.
4. Embrace life's challenges, and see the lessons to be learned.
5. Being blessed does not mean that your life is always bountiful and happy.
6. You can't control every aspect of your life, but you can control how you respond.
7. Life requires companionship. Seek the support and shelter of family and friends.
8. Be honest and emotionally vulnerable, and your relationships will flourish.
9. Laugh.
10. Laugh some more.

Time is
Too Slow for those who Wait,
Too Swift for those who Fear,
Too Long for those who Grieve,
Too Short for those who Rejoice,
But for those who Love,
Time is Eternity.
—Henry Van Dyke

Postscript

The transplant journey is a very perilous undertaking; it offers no guarantees or promises. As of July 2003, there are 3,885 people who are currently waiting for lungs, and of that number, only 1,000 people will receive the gift of life this year. Annually, approximately 432 people die nationwide waiting for lungs that will never come, and for those fortunate enough to receive a lung, 12 percent of them will die within the first three months, and 50 percent will be dead at the end of five years.

Despite these odds, the waiting list for lungs continues to grow each year because there is hope in transplantation: a dream of a new reality and a new vigor. A lung transplant can be a remarkably transformational process in which individuals who were once confined are miraculously able to live and breathe again. Human beings cling to life, and they cling to hope. Even in our darkest hours, we hold fast to the belief that we can somehow, someway beat the odds.

Doug and I are acutely aware that his transplant will continue to be a journey of challenges, sadness, beauty, and joy. It is simply the journey of life that we all must endure. Life is hard, and although it offers no guarantees to anyone, it does allow each of us to dream about tomorrow's possibilities. Doug has already survived the first nine months, and I choose to believe that he will be alive at the end of five years. It is with that approach that Doug and I, strengthened by the knowledge that each day is a beautiful gift that is given by the grace of God, will head toward our proverbial sunset. It is our bittersweet chance.

Lots of people want to ride with you in the limo, but what you want is someone who will take the bus with you when the limo breaks down.

—Oprah Winfrey

Resources and Support

Cystic-L

CYSTIC-L is a free email service dedicated to the exchange of information and support specific to cystic fibrosis. Since 1994, CYSTIC-L has been sharing both casual banter about the varied impact that CF has on our lives, as well as technical and medical information exchanges that help us to overcome the more unpleasant factors that this gene imposes upon us. There are over 600 list subscribers sending a total of around 20-60 messages per day; a digest option is available which compiles messages and distributes them periodically during the day. Members include people with CF and those who share their lives: medical professionals, scientists, researchers, parents, grandparents, spouses, siblings, friends, and significant others. To subscribe send the following line in the "body" of an email (the "subject" line is ignored) to **LISTSERV@PEACH.EASE.LSOFT.COM** SUBSCRIBE CYSTIC-L Your-first-name Your-last-name

Second Wind

Second Wind Lung Transplant Association, Inc. was formed on April 17, 1995 by a small group of people that wanted to supply information about lung transplantation to others. In 1995 lung transplantation was truly the beginning of a new horizon in medical technology. The slogan "Support through Service" was adopted, as was our mission statement: To improve the quality of life for lung transplant recipients, lung surgery candidates, people with related pulmonary concerns and their families, by providing support, love, advocacy, education, information and guidance through a spirit of service, adding years to their lives and life to their years.

We are an international organization over 800 members strong, with members scattered throughout the United States, many relocating to other states during the transplantation process. Lung disease not only affects our members, but entire families as well.

The Second Wind Lung Transplant Association organizes a Semi-Annual Education Conference bringing in many world-renowned surgeons, healthcare professionals, and participants striving to educate and support the growing numbers of lung transplant recipients and candidates.

Second Wind has a very active mailing list of 300 subscribers on the internet. To subscribe, send an email to **listserv@home.ease.lsoft.com** in the body of an email: SUB SECONDWIND first name surname (NOTE: DO NOT use your e-mail address).

ConnColl

ConnColl is an online support group whose purpose is to disseminate information concerning cystic fibrosis, to give unconditional support to those involved with the disease, to provide a forum for the discussion of topics relative to cystic fibrosis, to give members the opportunity to have an exchange of their ideas and interests not directly related to cystic fibrosis, and to provide contact with others who have or have an interest in cystic fibrosis. Please subscribe at the following web address:**http://chestnut.conncoll.edu/mailman/listinfo/cysticfibrosis**

CF Roundtable and the USACFA

USACFA (United States Adult cystic fibrosis Association) was founded in 1990. It is a totally independent, non-profit, and tax-exempt organization that is comprised of adults who have cystic fibrosis and give their time and energy voluntarily. There are no paid employees. The purpose of USACFA is to provide a source of information and education for adults who have CF in regard to the basic nature and progression of the disease, the latest in research and treatments to fight the disease, and to assist in the psycho-social aspects of coping with the disease on a day-to-day basis. One way we do this is through our publication CF Roundtable.

CF Roundtable is published quarterly and provides a network for adults who have CF. It also facilitates communication between patients, families, friends, and those in the medical and research professions.

One of our goals is to reach every adult who has CF in the USA. Another is to provide a resource for support groups to receive information and be able to share it with their potential memberships.

USACFA is not affiliated with any other organization and depends solely on tax-deductible donations to survive. To receive CF Roundtable, we ask for an annual donation of $10 from individuals and $25 from institutions. Subscribers with addresses outside the USA are asked to donate $15 (US funds only) to help cover postage costs. CF Roundtable is free to all adults who have CF and are unable to afford a donation.

If you would like to receive CF Roundtable, please write to: USACFA, Inc., PO Box 1618, Gresham, OR 97030-0519.

Printed in the United States
27759LVS00003B/142-156

9 781413 713244